INTERMITTENT FASTING

FOR WOMEN OVER 50

The Ultimate Guide For Fast And Easy Weight Loss. Burning Fat For An Aging Woman, Support Hormones, Detox Body With Intermittent Fasting And Autophagy.

Table of Contents

INTRODUCTION 7

CHAPTER 1: WHAT IS INTERMITTENT FASTING? 8

AUTOPHAGY AND HOW INTERMITTENT FASTING CAN
IMPROVE IT...13

    Microautophagy...14

    Macroautophagy..15

20/4 INTERMITTENT FASTING 16

16:8 INTERMITTENT FASTING 17

THE 12/12 INTERMITTENT FASTING...21

CHAPTER 2: INTERMITTENT FASTING FOR WOMEN
OVER 50 24

CHAPTER 3: WHY INTERMITTENT FASTING IS IDEAL
FOR WOMEN OVER 50...31

IMPROVED MENTAL CONCENTRATION AND CLARITY 31

IMPROVEMENT IN HORMONE PROFILE 31

REDUCES INFLAMMATION 31

SUPPORTS HEALTHY BODILY FUNCTIONS 31

POLYCYSTIC OVARIAN SYNDROME AND INTERMITTENT
FASTING 32

METABOLIC RESET 32

CHANGE IN CELL FUNCTION 33

IMPROVED SLEEP 33

MOOD AND MOTIVATION... 33

CARDIOVASCULAR HEALTH 34

GUT HEALTH... 34

WEIGHT LOSS.. 34

LOWER THE RISK OF DIABETES... 35

IT BOOSTS YOUR METABOLIC RATE 35

CONVERT YOUR BODY FAT 35

IMPROVE MUSCLE HEALTH 36

BOOSTED ENERGY 36

REDUCE INSULIN RESISTANCE.. 37

INCREASE NEURAL CELLS.. 38

LESSEN OXIDATIVE STRESS 38

IMPROVE MENTAL WELL-BEING 39

TREAT OR PREVENT DISEASE 39
LESS FOOD CONSUMPTION 40
IT SLOWS DOWN THE PROGRESSION OF CANCER. 40
REDUCES INFLAMMATION.. 40
HEART'S HEALTH 41
CELLULAR REPAIR 41
SUPPORTS YOU IN HEALING FASTER 41
MAY EXTEND YOUR LIFESPAN 42
BOOSTS YOUR IMMUNE SYSTEM...42
IMPROVED SEX DRIVE 42
CELLULAR REPAIR 43
CHAPTER 4: PROS AND CONS OF INTERMITTENT
FASTING..44
    Pros of Intermittent Fasting 45
    Cons of Intermittent Fasting 49
CHAPTER 5: ENHANCING INTERMITTENT FASTING
FOR YOU...53
RESEARCH, RESEARCH, RESEARCH 53
UNDERSTAND YOUR MOTIVATION 53
SLOW AND STEADY WINS THE RACE...54
DRINK PLENTY OF WATER 54
AVOID TEMPTATION 55
ENJOY THE CAFFEINE BOOST 56
STAY BUSY 56
LIBERALLY SEASON YOUR FOOD 57
PRIORITIZE HIGH-QUALITY AND CONSISTENT SLEEP 57
TRACK YOUR PROGRESS..58
AVOID FASTING WHEN STRESSED 59
CHAPTER 6: WEIGHT LOSS AND HEALTHY LIVING 60
CAUSE OF WEIGHT GAIN... 60
A HEALTHY AND BALANCED DIET 62
REGULATING YOUR METABOLISM..64
HOW TO USE FASTING FOR WEIGHT LOSS...................................64
CHAPTER 7: BREAKFAST 65
ZUCCHINI OMELET 66
CHILI OMELET.. 68
BASIL AND CHERRY TOMATO BREAKFAST..................................70

CARROT BREAKFAST SALAD 72
GARLIC ZUCCHINI MIX 74
CRUSTLESS BROCCOLI SUN-DRIED TOMATO QUICHE 75
CHOCOLATE PANCAKES 77
BREAKFAST SCRAMBLE 79
OATMEAL 81
COCONUT CREAM WITH BERRIES.. 82
SEAFOOD OMELET 83
SPINACH AND PORK WITH FRIED EGGS 85
SMOKED SALMON SANDWICH 87
SHRIMP DEVILED EGGS 90
SCRAMBLED EGGS WITH HALLOUMI CHEESE............................ 92
COCONUT PORRIDGE 94
WESTERN OMELET 95
MUSHROOM OMELET 97
FRITTATA WITH FRESH SPINACH 99
CAULIFLOWER HASH BROWNS 101
SALMON FILLED AVOCADO 103
RUTABAGA FRITTERS WITH AVOCADO 105
BACON MUSHROOM BREAKFAST CASSEROLE 107
BAKED EGGS 109
KETO BLUEBERRY MUFFINS 110
TACO BREAKFAST SKILLET.. 112
CREAM CHEESE PANCAKES 114
KETO CLOUD BREAD.. 115
CHAPTER 8: LUNCH... 117
VEGAN TUNA SALAD 117
VEGGIE WRAP WITH APPLES AND SPICY HUMMUS...................... 119
TURMERIC RACK OF LAMB.. 121
SAUSAGE CASSEROLE 123
CAJUN PORK SLIDERS..125
MAC AND CHEESE BITES...127
CHICK'N SALAD WITH CRANBERRIES AND PISTACHIOS................. 129
TUNA CASSEROLE 131
WHITE FISH WITH CURRY AND COCONUT..............................133
CREAMY FISH CASSEROLE 135
SPINACH AND GOAT CHEESE PIE 137

AVOCADO PIE..139

TEX MEX STUFFED ZUCCHINI BOATS 141

BRUSSEL SPROUTS AND HAMBURGER GRATIN 143

SOYLIME ROASTED TOFU..145

CHICKEN NUGGETS..146

CRAB-STUFFED AVOCADO 148

THAI FISH CURRY 150

AVOCADO GRAPEFRUIT SALAD 151

GARLIC HERB GRILLED CHICKEN BREAST............................153

CAJUN SHRIMP 155

SESAME-CRUSTED MAHI-MAHI 157

COUNTRY CHICKEN...159

MAHI-MAHI TACOS WITH AVOCADO AND FRESH CABBAGE 161

CHAPTER 9: DINNER...163

PAN-FRIED JACKFRUIT OVER PASTA WITH LEMON COCONUT
CREAM SAUCE..163

BUTTERNUT SQUASH TACOS WITH TEMPEH CHORIZO..................166

COATED CAULIFLOWER HEAD..168

ARTICHOKE PETALS BITES 170

STUFFED BEEF LOIN IN STICKY SAUCE 172

VEGAN FISH STICKS AND TARTAR SAUCE 175

VEGAN PHILLY CHEESESTEAK...178

PIGS IN A BLANKET 180

BAKED FISH STICKS 182

LEMON PARMESAN BAKED COD 184

BACON-WRAPPED MEATLOAF...186

ASIAN MEATBALLS WITH BASIL SAUCE.................................188

KORMA CURRY...190

ZUCCHINI BARS 192

MUSHROOM SOUP 194

STUFFED PORTOBELLO MUSHROOMS....................................196

LETTUCE SALAD...198

ONION SOUP 200

ASPARAGUS SALAD..202

CHAPTER 10: 4 WEEKS MEAL PLAN 204

CONCLUSION 207

Introduction

In this book, we will talk about intermittent fasting, more specifically on how someone should follow intermittent fasting if they are above the age of 50.

Many people don't realize it, but intermittent fasting is fantastic for people who are above the age of 50 as it helps them to slow down aging and detoxify their bodies. One of the main things to worry about once you get up to the age of 50 is that you need body while healing the body the right way so that you can slow down the aging process. Who doesn't want to live for a very long time and to be healthy at the same time? Everybody wants to achieve this goal, which is why we have written this book so that many people who are looking to slow down aging or to feel better about themselves can read along and change their life. Couple things to remember before you start implementing and reading this book, make sure that you consult with your doctor before you begin any plan. The truth is we don't know what situation you are in, which is why we recommend that you consult with a professional before you start intermittent fasting as it cannot be ideal for everyone. Another thing to remember would be that intermittent fasting has to be done correctly, so make sure that you understand everything in this book before you start implementing the tips and tricks. Other than that, you should be good to go when it comes to intermittent fasting.

Chapter 1:
What Is Intermittent Fasting?

In this chapter, we will talk about intermittent fasting and what it means to follow intermittent fasting. If you have been living under a rock, there's a high chance that you have no idea what intermittent fasting is or what it can do for you. What we will do is go through the basics of intermittent fasting so that you understand what intermittent fasting is and that you have a better understanding of it moving on.

The problem with modern-day and fad diets is that it is simply not sustainable in the long-term. If you want to lose weight and feel better by yourself for the rest of your life, then you need to pick something which is not only sustainable but can be adjusted into your lifestyle based on your needs. Moreover, you need something that gives you the freedom to eat and have whatever it is that you like in moderation so that you can enjoy life and be with your friends and family a lot more often. The truth is, many fad diets do not allow you to eat food, which is unhealthy. Don't get me wrong; eating unhealthy food all the time is not the best thing for your body anyways.

However, we recommend that you eat decent quality food often so that you see the benefits that you are looking for when it comes to losing fat or building muscle. However, eating decent food all the time can be a tedious task, which can lead to failure in the long-term, which is why having unhealthy food which tastes good here and there can lead to overall success in the long-term. With that being said, following fat diets play does not allow you to eat anything which is unhealthy. Most of the time, the fad diets put you in a position where you are insanely starving your body. Starving your body in the short-term might lead to weight loss, which might make you feel better, however starving yourself in the long-term can lead to many unwanted health fallbacks.

This is another reason why people who start following fad diets tend to give up so soon. This is where intermittent fasting comes in; the great thing about intermittent fasting is that many people don't even switch up what they are eating. What they do is eat cyclically. They would eat for certain hours of the day and would not eat for certain hours of the day. In essence, intermittent fasting is a cyclical way of eating. Now the most common way for people to follow intermittent fasting would be the 16/8 method. And this method you will be eating for 8 hours of the day, and you will be fasting for 16 hours of the day.

This is where you will not get any food to eat, and we'll have to survive on water or black coffee. You can have anything you want, which has no calories when you are fasting. Now there are tons of intermittent fasting methods which we will talk about later on in this book. However, the 16/8 method has been working very well for most people and can be added to their lifestyle. The great thing about this method would be that you don't have to worry about having certain hours to be more important than others when it comes to eating window and visa-versa. You will be the one picking out the times for your eating window and your fasting window. The most common times for fasting are 8 pm till 12 pm the next day, then eating from 12 pm to 8 pm, again this time could be whatever works for your schedule.

Another great thing about intermittent fasting would be that there are no restrictions on what you could be eating. For example, during the eating window, many people eat whatever they want within reason to achieve their goals. I have seen many Fitness professionals eat food such as buttermilk biscuit, or even candy and dessert sometimes during the eating window, and still lose weight. We don't recommend you do that. However, this plan gives you the freedom to eat whatever you want while still seeing the results when it comes to losing fat and building muscle.

If you want to lose fat even more efficiently when intermittent fasting, we recommend that you eat a good, well-balanced diet slightly in a caloric deficit. This will allow you to not only lose fat but also to be certain that you're going to see results in the long-term when it comes to overall health and well-being. We also recommend that you accompany this with a fitness plan, make sure that you're working out in the gym if you want to lose fat and see the results that you have been hoping for. Another great thing about intermittent fasting, especially for people who are over the age of 50 years, is that it slows aging. One of the very best things, when it comes to intermittent fasting would be that it allows you to have very well-balanced aging and to make you look younger. These are thanks to two things, and the first one would be the increase in growth hormone. As you may know, intermittent fasting has shown to increase growth hormone production. This hormone is the youth of foundation, the reason why is because it will help you to recover quickly.

The benefits of growth hormone also include better skin and better bones, and you will also lose more fat and build more muscle. Another thing that intermittent fasting helps with would be the process known as autophagy. Autophagy is a process where your body gets rid of old/dead cells and replaces them with new cells.

This is the reason why you see the youth benefits, and also the reason why many people stay young for a very long time. These detoxifying cells would also mean getting rid of any diseased cells, which may include cancerous cells. Many people claim to get rid of their cancer very quickly by following intermittent fasting, and we can't back that up; however, it has been claimed by many cancer survivors. If you're someone looking to not only be better when it comes to Performance inside and outside the gym but also to look a lot younger in the long-term, then you have no reason why not to follow intermittent fasting. We will make it very easy for you when it comes to picking out the right plan and how to follow it appropriately.

Understand this, and intermittent fasting could be one of the easiest plans you could follow. And it all starts by reading this book. Do you have already taken the first step to seeing better results with your body and health, so make sure that you go all the way with it. Intermittent fasting is like eating in increments. As we told you, it is a cyclical way of eating food, which allows you to consume all the calories you need in a certain hour of the day. While certain of the day, you will be fasting and not eating anything at all. Once you start following intermittent fasting, you will be surprised how much time we spend on eating food. We spend a lot of time, more specifically waste a lot of time eating food. If you're someone who is looking to see success with their business or their work environment, then you will gain from that time and see the results that you have been hoping for. Intermittent fasting truly is a win-win situation. It makes you feel younger, and it gets rid of any bad cells in your body while increasing all the good hormones. Think of it this way, and there are many people who follow intermittent fasting without even knowing it. Many religions recommend that you fast for 30 days, or however long. This goes to show intermittent fasting has been in practice for a very long time, and good reason, it simply works.

Now, if you are someone who can't fast every day for the rest of your life, don't worry as you will have at least one day in the week or you can eat throughout the whole day. We recommend that you do that as it will allow you to be more motivated in the long-term, which is what intermittent fasting is all about is creating a lifestyle. If you are tired of following diets that yield you some results, but they aren't sustainable in the long-term, then chances are intermittent fasting is going to be your savior.

Make sure that you pick the plan that fits your needs and your goals. We will talk about all the intermittent fasting methods later on in this book. However, once you understand the benefits and the reasons why you need to be following intermittent fasting, then it will be straightforward for you to follow it in the long-term. The main thing that differentiates intermittent fasting to any other fad diet is that they're health benefits to intermittent fasting and not just aesthetic benefits. Meaning, God guides give you a set of promises which may or may not be delivered. However, intermittent fasting has shown time and time again to deliver aesthetic benefits, and on top of that, help you get rid of many diseases that will help you stay healthy for a very long time.

Intermittent fasting is also one of the best plans to follow up for someone who's over the age of 50. The reasons why we told you is because it helps you to say younger and to enjoy life a lot more when you're 50 the main thing you want to do is enjoy the life, if you want to enjoy life then you need to be in a healthy State of Mind and Body. Intermittent fasting gives you all of that, and on top of that, it helps you to say a lot younger for a very long time. If you don't believe me, then look at your celebrities, many celebrities who are in their 50s tend to follow intermittent fasting and for an excellent reason. It is because it helps them to stay younger and to think a lot better and quickly.

Finally, intermittent fasting helps you to save a lot more time because you will not be thinking about eating for a certain amount of time, which will allow you to spend that time working on your craft. With that being said, we now conclude this chapter.

Autophagy and How Intermittent Fasting Can Improve It

Autophagy is one of the most powerful cleaning processes carried out by the body. Recently, a Japanese scientist Dr. Yoshinori Oshumi won the Nobel peace prize in 2016 for his research on the concept. He found that the body had a very unique ability to purge all the bad elements in the body including the "misformed" proteins, pathogens, and unwanted infections that are harming the body if it senses an acute shortage of energy. This means that if a person is starving, the body would turn off all the bad process in the body and would start using them to produce energy. It would become a highly efficient machine to survive for the longest.

At the heart of intermittent fasting's benefits is the science that makes all of it work. Autophagy is the biological process in which your cells, when unable to get energy from food, consume "junk" materials such as unused organelles, proteins, and foreign toxins.

You put your body through autophagy when you do intermittent fasting because you are depriving your cells of food to consume, so they switch to autophagy to get their energy. Because of this, you can reap all the advantages of autophagy by simply not eating during certain windows of the day.

Even if you are a fan of learning about science, it is easy to get overwhelmed with information overload, especially when you only learned about autophagy recently. But there are some simple facts that will make things easier for you. Firstly, I am not leaving out anything important in this chapter. You can rest easy knowing that you are not missing something important about autophagy in this chapter.

Part of the reason learning the science behind intermittent fasting is so important is because you need to be certain of autophagy's significance yourself. If you can't tell your friends in a few sentences why you are doing intermittent fasting, you will lose sight of the purpose of it, and you might be in danger of stopping. You will have more than a few sentences to say to back up the science of intermittent fasting after reading this chapter. It is probable that you might annoy your friends with facts about autophagy for a week or so after reading.

They might be annoyed with you, but they won't be able to discredit the points your making, so you will probably be doing their health a favor. Doing intermittent fasting is a lot more fun when you have friends or family doing it with you, so learning the ins and outs of the science behind intermittent fasting is a great opportunity to recruit others to help you live more healthily.

Microautophagy

This is the form that autophagy takes in every single cell of your body. All cells have lysosomes, and those lysosomes have the chief purpose of conducting microautophagy. As usual, their job is to bring in damaged organelles to break them down. This is different from macroautophagy and chaperone-mediated autophagy, where the lysosome does not pull in the cellular waste on its own. In those kinds of autophagy, a special organelle called the autophagosome has the job of finding waste inside and outside of the cell. Then, it carries them over to the lysosome and binds with it to break down its contents.

Microautophagy happens in every cell because it does some very important jobs. It helps with the homeostasis of the membrane and it keeps the cell's organelles at their current size.

The chemical function of the lysosome is still being studied, but essentially its method of breaking down the cellular waste is attacking them with enzymes. Finally, microautophagy is finished and the cell uses the raw materials attained from breaking down the waste for its part of the cell cycle. The cell can use the materials for building a new cell, building a new organelle, or for building even more basic things like glucose, amino acids, fatty acids, and so forth.

Macroautophagy

Macroautophagy is the type of autophagy that is only seen in cells with certain jobs. This type and chaperone-mediated autophagy use the autophagosome. The autophagosome can be simply described as a vesicle — that is, it can carry things inside of it and transport them. This vesicle (the autophagosome) travels around inside the cell and goes outside the cell to find waste to break down when you are fasting, and food is scarce. When it is done wandering through the cytoplasm finding waste, it returns to the lysosome and binds with it.

When the autophagosome takes the materials into the lysosome, this is called sequestration. The autophagosome has a double membrane around it that it uses to trap materials inside. When sequestration occurs, both membranes open so that the lysosome can take the toxins that the vesicle found. But in macroautophagy, it is not the lysosome that breaks down the toxins, but the autophagosome. It can only break them down when it is bonded to the lysosome, however.

Since macroautophagy only happens in specialized cells like white blood cells, there are actually a few different kinds of macroautophagy itself, such as mitophagy and ribophagy. Most of the time, these different kinds of macroautophagy are made for getting rid of specific organelles that have stopped working.

This process can also be used for great advantage as it gives the unique opportunity to get rid of most of the diseases. Even the progression of scariest diseases like cancer can be slowed down with by inducing autophagy. To initiate autophagy, you do not need to do anything extra. You simply need to stop adding anything extra to your body and the process would begin on its own.

Fasting is the only way through which autophagy can begin. Studies have further shown that although long fasts are more effective in initiating autophagy, it can also begin with fasts as small as 12-14 hours every day. This means that by following intermittent fasting you can get the unique advantages of autophagy.

Autophagy is the ultimate solution for most of the diseases in the body. It has the ability to treat diseases and bring longevity. You would feel younger and healthier if your body is going through autophagy. It is the process in which your body is utilizing all the waste products to produce energy and cells. Nothing gets wasted and every resource is put to best use.

Intermittent fasting opens the doors of holistic health for you. It makes staying healthy and fit very easy without having to go through the torturous routine of elaborate diets that don't even give you enough to eat. You wouldn't have to keep feeling restricted and desperate through the whole process as eating some of the things becomes a dream. Intermittent fasting will give you great freedom and ease of life. You will simply have to follow some basic rules and the doors of good health will open for you without having to spend large sums of money or time.

20/4 Intermittent fasting

While a more extreme version of fasting, women who have adjusted to the 16/8 fasting method and want more of a challenge may desire to try the 20/4 fast. A large fluid intake must accompany the twenty hours of fasting during the fasting window. During your four-hour eating window, try to eat two large and calorie-dense meals, full of healthy nutrients. You will want these meals to contain your entire caloric, protein, and fat needs for the day.

This fast is often best started after lunchtime. By starting after lunch, you can enjoy a large breakfast, lunch, and maybe even a snack before you begin your fast. If you finish lunch at 12 pm, then your fast will go until the following day at 8 am, meaning you can eat your meals that day as usual.

If you find this fast is overly tricky when you first start, don't hesitate to cut it short. Instead of pushing yourself to finish the full twenty-hour fast, you can slowly increase your fasting window naturally until you get to your goal.

16:8 Intermittent fasting

As is it in the name, this method involves two periods, a 16-hour fasting period and an 8-hour period of eating. It is advisable to keep your feeding periods constant to make the body it easy for your body to adapt and make it easy to follow. You cannot switch the feeding times around, as you want every day. Ghrelin, the hunger hormone, is released in according to your eating pattern. Constant changing of your eating pattern with mess with your hormones and leave you feeling hungry all the time.

16/8 Fasting Protocol Over 24 Hours

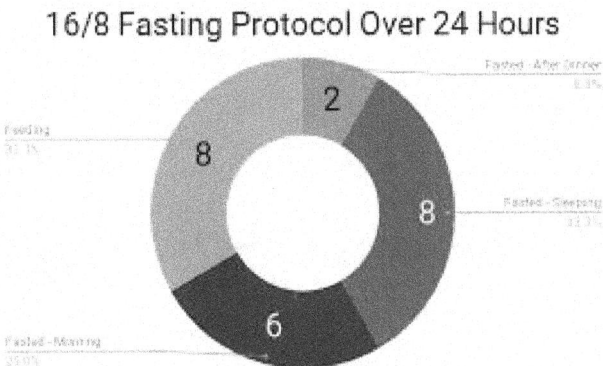

It is a very sustainable and easy to keep on doing since you do not go long without food and can fit into your schedule effortlessly. This is also because part of the period when your fasting is at night, so the fasting period seems shorter. An example of the 16:8 schedule is if you eat at 10 pm, you will fast until 2 pm the following day.

It is true that your body will get used to being in a fasted state, but the journey to that point is not that easy, as you will be going against your body's food desires. These craving will be most powerful in the first two weeks but will greatly reduce after. So how do you deal with these cravings and keep on fasting?

Set clear goals that you want to achieve. What do you aim to accomplish with this fasting regiment? As it gets tougher, goals like wanting to get fit, health or burn some fat will not motivate you at all. If you do not have a clear reason for doing a fast, you are more likely to quit than someone who has specific goals. You should know what you want to achieve soon and in the long run. How do you want to look in 2 months? How do you want to feel in 5 months? What do you want your health to be like in 12 months? All these and more are the questions you should be asking yourself. Even after knowing what you want in those time periods, you should also ask yourself the reason for wanting those things and the effect of the objective to your life if it is achieved. This helps you to see things in a way that is more relevant to you. If you have the urge to eat that extra piece of cake, remember how in the end, if you achieve your goal, your life will change.

Make it a point to know why you are craving a certain food. Is it because of actual thirst and hunger because of boredom? Are you just tired or stressed and looking for comfort in food? Try your best to distract yourself so that you do not end up eating during your fasting period. You should always give yourself-hope that you will make it through the craving period. It will pass, it always does.

Different things, in this book we will only talk about food, tempt us all at times. Removing temptation foods from your house will make it a lot easier to not be tempted to eat them.

If following recipes too tough at first, you can substitute them with shakes as you get used to it.

Organize your schedule. You may choose an eating window and discover that you do not have time to eat at that time. Do not set your eating window at a time you know it will be hard to go without food like if you eat when you are bored then don't set your eating period during the slowest part of the day. If you have, a meal with your family at a certain time then put your eating window at that time. Make wise choices when deciding your feeding window. It always best to make it as easy as possible for you to follow.

Be your own support pillar. When you are starving, there is always this voice in your head that gives you many reasons why it is good to break your diet. It happens to us all when we are vulnerable. It is important for you to not listen to that voice. Even if you break the fast just once, you will eventually do it repeatedly. It is best to stay strong. If you give in, it happens to even the best of fasters, then do not use it as an excuse to stop fasting completely, keep on going because you only truly fail when you stop trying.

On top of personal support, also external support can help you. Make it a point to be around positive people who are on the same path as you. It will get hard and quitting will seem like the only option but if you have other people supporting you, it will keep you going. The more the better, you will be able to support each other, and you will all eventually reach your targets.

Stay hydrated. Dehydration sometimes may be interpreted as hunger by the body. Sometimes you might think that you are hungry while in actual sense you are just thirsty. Drink lots of water, black coffee, sparkling water, black tea or any other drink, which has zero calories.

Be patient. You may think of intermittent fasting as the magic bullet you can use to burn all your fat instantly but that is not possible. All good things take time, so does burning fat. You cannot workout and fast for two days and expect to have lost many pounds, do not get frustrated. You will only be able to see good results if you remain consistent through the process.

 Give your body time to adapt to fasting. No living organism accepts change easily, your body will have to get used to the new way of life you have chosen and can react differently to fewer meals. Among the possible discomforts are headaches, hunger, and even body weakness. Better direction than speed, you might be moving slowly but in the right direction or you can be moving at supersonic speed in the wrong one. Do not give up.

One of the major factors that can help you succeed in intermittent fasting, which is overlooked by many, is sleep. The importance of sleep is not given enough weight by many books and articles on 16:8 intermittent fasting. Proper sleep can boost your overall fasting results by a large percentage. When you sleep, our bodies repair the damage, burn fat and replace cells. In sleep, both the quality and the quantity matter.

There are various ways of improving the quality of your sleep. First, get more sunlight. You "body clock" does not understand time the same way you do, it knows the time by light signals. Sunlight heavily influences it. Morning sunlight signals your glands and organs to wake up and make them produce hormones that should be used in the day. If you get a little sunlight in the day and on top of that, a lot of artificial light in the night, our circadian clock gets messed up. This malfunction can make your body produce hormones that can prevent you from sleeping. If you do not get enough quality sleep, there can be an increase in hormones such as insulin and hindrance to the production of hormones such as HGH causing no fat to be burnt at night.

You should also make it a point to avoid screens before bedtime. If you fall asleep watching TV or using your phone, it is best to keep away from them. Your body clock is not only affected by sunlight but also artificial light. These screens mostly produce blue light, which makes our body produce hormones that were meant to keep you awake and active. Falling asleep will be hard. Do not make it a habit of sleeping while using these devices. It is best to sleep in darkness. It is easier to sleep that way plus it can help you sleep better. Blackout your windows or put up heavy-duty curtains if there are annoying streetlights and other outside light sources that you cannot control.

There is a certain period in the night as you sleep that your body produces the best number of hormones required for fat burning and repair. It is best, if possible, to get into bed as once darkness falls. Healthy life, weight loss, and muscle building are just some of the many benefits of improving your sleeping habits. It may even do more than increasing the hours you spend in the gym.

The 12/12 Intermittent fasting

This intermittent fast is a good one to start with, although if the idea of fasting is completely new to you and makes you nervous, you are totally free to reduce it to 10 hours or less.

The trick for a simple intermittent fast like this is to ensure you are still getting the healthy number of calories every day but to simply get them outside of the 12-hour long window that you have decided to fast for.

The 12-hour fast is also a good place to start for someone who wants to end up doing a more ambitious fast. You don't start so low that going as high as 16 hours seems infeasible. You may even want to work up to a 20-hour fast if you are feeling bold, though, at that point, you may want to consider trying the 24-hour water fast.

The times during which you fast are entirely up to you. Any intermittent fast is best done by waking up relatively early, eating breakfast, fasting, and then eating dinner not too soon before bed. You don't want to eat too close to your bedtime because then you will be spending a lot of your precious autophagy time during sleep by breaking down your food.

It is surprising that we have not even had the opportunity to talk about the importance of sleep with autophagy. There are some facts about sleep and autophagy that you need to seriously consider.

You do the most autophagy that you do throughout your day when you are sleeping. Even in people who do not think about fasting or autophagy whatsoever, their highest level of autophagy is when they are sleeping, and so is yours.

That means when you eat really close to the time you go to bed — let's say you eat at 7pm and then sleep at 9pm — you aren't giving your body enough time to break down your food. You don't have any significant autophagy when you are digesting, so digesting in your sleep is a big wasted opportunity.

Even the 12-hour fast can prove challenging, because you don't want to wake up too unreasonably early, but you don't want to digest food during the time that you should be going through advanced autophagy while you are asleep, either.

You may choose to wake up and eat your first meal at 7am. 12 hours later, your fast is over, and you eat dinner at 7pm. You can probably already see how this can problematic; if you get enough sleep to wake up at 7am, you will want to be in bed by 10pm. However, this does leave 3 hours between your dinner and your bedtime, so while it is a tight squeeze, this system does work out for the 12-hour fast.

Chapter 2:
Intermittent Fasting for
Women over 50

Overweight women over 50 have a higher risk of diabetes and heart problems than they did when they were younger. IF is one option they have to manage their weight and control these health risks.

The metabolism of a woman over 50 has become slower, so you can't expect quick results if you are a member of this group, but you will probably get the most out of it than any other group of women because of all the anti-aging effects of IF and autophagy.

Overweight and obese people have higher risks of heart disease, stroke, and more as they age. On the other hand, thinner people are not looking at these same risks.

Losing weight can only be good for your body, and autophagy is the healthiest and most effective way to do it. Autophagy will help you stay thin, feel good, and be healthy for years and years.

But, so far, we have only talked about the health benefits that are immediately obvious. There is also a reduction of health risks that are not cosmetic like youthful skin and weight loss. It has been proven that an increase in autophagy reduces your risk of Alzheimer's and Parkinson's disease.

More autophagy also reduces inflammation, which will increase your overall health. There has even been research about the benefits of autophagy for cancer patients undergoing chemotherapy.

Studies have shown that cancer patients going through chemotherapy saw a reduction in the clumps of white blood cells that accumulate because of chemotherapy. Dead cells can be hazardous to your body if they are not cleaned out during autophagy.

Since these patients fasted in order to turn on autophagy, their bodies were able to clean out the white blood cells and recover from chemotherapy sooner.

You can only imagine the kind of advantage you get if you are turning autophagy on as much as possible, and you aren't even looking at a major health risk yet. You may not have as big an accumulation of dead cells as someone going through chemotherapy, but if you have not fasted before and you don't exercise regularly, it is very likely that you have a lot of toxins in your body.

This is because if you don't go through autophagy very often, materials like dead cells, dead organelles, and unused proteins start to pile up and make your cells less efficient.

Putting your body through autophagy doesn't just combat aging in ways that are immediately visible. It also greatly reduces your risk of long-term age-related disease. Whether you're looking to improve the quality of your life or the length of your life, making autophagy happen in your body will do it.

There are many misconceptions about how autophagy does its anti-aging work. Perhaps the most common is that its only health benefits come from taking care of toxins. Clearing toxins from your system is certainly a good thing, but autophagy goes far beyond ridding your body of harmful chemicals.

Most of these toxins are not from outside your body, but they are materials like proteins and organelles that your cells used once and then no longer had a use for. These discarded materials start to take up space over time, creating clutter that slows down your cells. This is when they become toxins.

Some of these toxins cause even worse problems than congestion. The worst case is protein clusters that form in the brain. Neurodegenerative diseases like Alzheimer's become more of a concern as we age, and autophagy might be your best ally in fighting against your risk of these diseases.

From a broader perspective, Alzheimer's manifests as "knots" and "tangles" in the brain that impair memory.

When doctors look at the knots and tangles with a microscope, they see that these irregularities are actually clusters of proteins that have built up over time. They are proteins that brain cells used at one point but later had no purpose. The protein clusters were not managed with autophagy, so they simply accumulated and started leading to serious memory problems.

Alzheimer's disease is the most extreme consequence that you can have from not going through enough autophagy. It is not the only consequence, however. Discarded materials like protein clusters start to build up throughout your body if you rarely go through autophagy.

In this regard, low autophagy leads to a low count of collagen, the protein that makes your skin youthful. Your skin cells can't produce collagen when they are crowded by cellular garbage.

Similarly, you lose more muscle mass if you rarely go through autophagy because you are not turning on autophagy to repair the muscle tissue damage that results from physical activity.

From these examples alone, you can see that autophagy is more than a toxin-cleaning agent. Autophagy doesn't only destroy the bad (toxins); it builds the good (new organelles, proteins, and cells). Both sides of autophagy make it such a powerful anti-aging tool, one that was surprisingly given to us by nature.

So far, we have established that autophagy isn't just good for destroying pathogen invaders — it also destroys materials that become toxic when they linger in the cell for too long. In short, this biological process cleans out toxins from the outside and inside.

In the third stage, your cells use these broken-down parts as ingredients to build new cells and cell structures. What's more: your cells have more room to build new cells and new cell parts because they freed up so much space during autophagy.

All these things come together when you find a way to turn on autophagy on a regular basis. Equipped with all this information, you know much more about autophagy than even your average fasting practitioner.

Women over 50 certainly still want to manage their weight and have good skin, but it is around this age that we start to get a more mature perspective on life, and we care more about the health consequences of our daily life choices than before. They have many options for unlocking autophagy even further than they would with IF alone.

Back in the 90s, the idea of caloric restriction became very popular, and people saw improvements in their health from doing nothing more than eating less. There is even a great deal of evidence that mammals who restrict their calories live longer than mammals who do not.

This has not yet been proven to be true for humans, but still, restricting your caloric intake can only be a good thing. You get this additional benefit from turning on autophagy through fasting while also getting the benefit of autophagy itself along with it.

We have heard a lot of ideas about losing weight from nutritionists in the last few decades, but let's not kid ourselves: the main reason for weight gain across the planet comes down to people consuming a lot of calories without physically exerting themselves to burn them off. Fasting for any length of time will lead to consuming fewer calories, so you are on the right track for losing weight when you fast.

The next popular method of turning on autophagy is the keto diet. This method will turn on autophagy because it involves depriving your body of nutrients that it would normally consume for energy.

However, following the keto diet alone will not turn on autophagy because it is only activated when your cells are in a state of stress, and as long as you are sedentary or filling your body with any kind of food, your cells are not in this state.

That said, since the keto diet is so low in carbs, this style of eating will aid in turning on autophagy. I definitely recommend following the keto diet because the mistake many autophagy practitioners make is consuming a lot of carbs while they are not fasting.

Eating a lot of carbs will prevent your body from fasting for a long time because it takes a long time for your digestive system to process them. Not only that, but as you may be aware, it becomes harder to keep weight off the older you get, and you are significantly slowing down the process of burning fat when your digestive tract has a backlog of carbs. Fighting against this problem is the role of the keto diet in anti-aging and autophagy.

Next, there is the method of good old exercise. Studies have shown that resistance training, also known as strength training, is the most effective way of turning on autophagy, saying it is even more effective than fasting. The reason for this is that when you use your muscles, you are getting tiny tears in your muscle tissue that are repaired through autophagy.

The unfortunate thing is that exercising might be the last thing that people want to do, even though it is so good for their health. Like the other methods, exercise has its own health benefits that are separate from autophagy.

Plenty of studies show that people who work out regularly have lower risks of all age-related illnesses, even those not related to the heart. If we are being honest, exercising is probably the best way to fight aging.

If you want to get the most out of autophagy, you should employ all of these methods together. When combined, the keto diet, exercise, and fasting will give you the greatest benefits, both in terms of weight loss and in general health.

If you don't yet feel motivated to be as healthy as possible, try to think of the autophagy in your cells as an analogy for your personal health. If they did not recycle their cellular garbage, your cells would simply die after their organelles stopped working or they were overcrowded with protein clusters and foreign invaders.

If you do not recycle your body's toxins by turning on autophagy regularly, your body will be over-encumbered with cellular garbage and you will be less healthy as a result. If this analogy were expanded, you might even live a shorter life if you do not regularly clean out your cellular garbage via autophagy.

Your cells try to live longer by using autophagy to combat their cellular aging — you should try to use autophagy to work against aging too.

Chapter 3:
Why Intermittent Fasting is Ideal for Women over 50

Improved Mental Concentration and Clarity

Fasting has incredible benefits for the healthy function of the brain. The most known benefit stems from the activation of autophagy, which is a cell cleansing process. Note that fasting has anti-seizure effects.

Improvement in Hormone Profile

There are plenty of people who avoid intermittent fasting as they feel it will cause their fitness levels to deteriorate. This isn't necessarily the case for those people who do take part in intermittent fasting, as studies have shown that fasting does not negatively impact those who perform regular physical activities, especially if you cut down on your carbs as you fast and are in a ketosis state. Studies have shown that physical training while fasting can lead to higher metabolic adaptations.

Reduces Inflammation

Intermittent fasting promotes autophagy, a process in which the body destroys its old or damaged cells. Killing off old cells may sound like a terrible notion. However, it can be seen as a way of removing old and unwanted dirt from your body. It's a simple method for the body to clean and repair itself. Old and damaged cells can create inflammation. Because intermittent fasting stimulates autophagy, then it is possible to reduce inflammation in your body while fasting.

Supports Healthy Bodily Functions

Intermittent fasting gives your body time to complete processes and functions before introducing more food into your system.

This means that every time you eat, you are giving your body adequate time to actually metabolize the food and use it appropriately. In modern society, we regularly overeat and push our bodies to constantly be in a state of digesting. As a result, our systems become overwhelmed and we do not effectively metabolize everything. This can lead to you not getting enough nutrition, storing fats, and struggling to produce healthy levels of natural hormones and chemicals within your body.

Polycystic Ovarian Syndrome and Intermittent Fasting

Polycystic ovaries are a fairly common disease in women. This disease causes a hormone shift and can have any undesirable effects on women. Many women struggle with weight gain and difficulty losing weight as a side effect of the disease. While there are not very many studies about how intermittent fasting affects the disease, there is evidence that combining intermittent fasting with a keto diet significantly helped to regulate the hormones and made weight loss possible for polycystic ovarian syndrome patients. There does seem to be some potential hope with using intermittent fasting to help treat and maintain diseases like polycystic ovarian syndrome and other hormonal disorders. Time and additional research will tell us if intermittent fasting has a future in helping with this disease.

Metabolic Reset

Many women, as they age, experience reduced metabolism. This is partly due to the natural aging process, and partly due to damaging the metabolism over the decades. Frequent crash dieting, poor sleep, overworking, poor health, and more can all damage your metabolism, thus preventing you from losing weight. But, by merely practicing intermittent fasting, you can reset and boost your metabolism, not only allowing you to lose weight but also helping you to feel healthier and maintain healthy lean muscle as you age.

Change in Cell Function

When you fast for a while, different changes take place in your body. For instance, your body will start a process of cellular repair and there will be changes in your hormone level. A difference in these levels makes it easier for the body to access the stored fat. You will notice that there is a reduction in the level of insulin and it helps increase the body's ability to burn fat. An increase in the human growth hormone helps to increase lean muscle and burn more fat than usual. Damaged cells are processed and other processes of cellular repair kick in. In addition, several changes take place within the genes and molecules that protect you against disease.

Improved Sleep

There has been at least one scientific study which has shown that people who persist with intermittent fasting for a year or more have better sleep. The reasons why this occurs are no doubt complicated, but there's been conclusive demonstrations that intermittent fasting over an extended period assists good sleep.

Mood and Motivation

The study of the effect of intermittent fasting on mood and motivation is in its infancy. There is a lack of research on large populations, using the statistical techniques of randomized controls. However, some studies have demonstrated that intermittent fasting does improve both mood and motivation in a surprisingly short period. As there is profound controversy about the pharmacological treatments of people's mental state, any treatment which has no side effects and many potential benefits must be considered seriously.

Cardiovascular Health

Intermittent fasting leads to a reduction in weight. For this and other reasons, it leads to an improvement in cardiovascular health. The cause of such disease is usually atherosclerosis, the deposit of plaque in blood vessel walls. The dysfunction of the endothelium, which is a thin lining of the blood vessels, causes atherosclerosis. A healthy endothelium works to prevent this insidious deposit. The endothelium is not doing its job properly if plaque builds up. Obesity, especially where the fat deposits are in the abdominal area, leads in many cases to this buildup of plaque.

Other causes of this deposit are stress and inflammation. Intermittent fasting assists in the reduction of these, as well as obesity. Some studies show improvements in all risk factors for cardiovascular health.

Gut Health

Increasingly, scientists are becoming ever more aware that microorganisms living in the human gut or digestive system perform vital functions. These are known as the microbiome. There are trillions of them and they are in other parts of the body, apart from the gut. Many diseases originate in the gut, not only illnesses concerning that part of the body, but also of the brain, the heart, and all other regions of the body.

There is research on mice that caloric restriction improves that part of the microbiome in the gut. The effect of this is to prolong the life of the mice. In humans, the effects of dietary changes are very swift, even as short as hours. Studies are currently being done to verify that the real effects of intermittent fasting observed in the gut health of mice are true for humans as well.

Weight Loss

The most obvious benefit of this diet is weight loss. When you follow intermittent fasting, the number of meals you eat will be reduced. When you eat less, the calories you consume will decrease as well. When the levels of insulin decline, growth hormone increases along with an increase in norepinephrine, which helps the body break down stored fat to provide energy. There is an increase in your metabolic rate when you fast, which helps the body burn more calories. The effect of intermittent fasting is two-fold. On the one hand, it increases your metabolic rate and therefore makes your body more efficient while burning fats. The reduction in the level of food you consume reduces your overall calorie intake.

Lower the Risk of Diabetes

The most common health problem that plagues humanity these days, apart from obesity, is diabetes. High blood sugar leads to insulin resistance in the body. Intermittent fasting helps to reduce blood sugar and therefore helps reduce insulin resistance in the body. When your body becomes resistant to insulin, it leads to an increase in the blood sugar level and the vicious cycle goes on and on. If you opt for this diet, you can successfully reverse this condition.

It boosts your metabolic rate

Studies show that staying in a fasted state leads to a spike in the hormone norepinephrine. This hormone increases your basal metabolic rate and burns fat. On top of that, once you enter your eating window, your metabolism still stays at an elevated level. You are essentially burning excess fat even when eating!

Convert Your Body Fat

Many people are unaware, but there are two types of body fat, white and brown. This fat is not created equal. Just as there is healthy and unhealthy cholesterol, there is also sturdy and unhealthy body fat. The white fat, which is what builds up as people gain excess weight, is damaging to health, contributes to aging, and leads to disease.

On the other hand, brown body fat is vital in protecting the body's inner organs and maintaining health. When you practice intermittent fasting, it not only helps you lose weight, but it can also actively convert your unhealthy white fat to healthy brown fat. As if that weren't good enough, brown fat also helps burn off white fat, meaning that the more brown fat you have, the more you will burn off excess white body fat.

Improve Muscle Health

Many people get excited about the temporary weight reduction they experience when trying the crash diet. That is until they stop losing weight and eventually give up on a diet. But, most of the weight loss people achieve on these diets is not fat loss but water weight and muscle weight. Muscle weighs more than fat, so even a small amount of muscle loss can make a big difference on the scale.

As crash diets promote malnutrition, it naturally leads to muscle loss, which negatively affects your health and strength as you age. After all, your muscles are in much more than your arms. They are surrounding your entire body, and even your heart is a muscle! As you lose muscle, your health and energy will be dramatically affected, and it is essential to regain this as you age if you want to improve your health. Thankfully, studies have found that when compared to dieting, intermittent fasting not only leads to more weight loss than dieting, but it also causes much less muscle loss. This means your muscles will become much healthier, especially if you actively workout while you practice fasting.

Boosted Energy

The mitochondria, which are within our mitochondrial cells, are the powerhouse of the cell. It is the mitochondria that allow us to use a variety of fuel sources from the food we eat as fuel, as well as ketones. While other cells in the body may only be able to utilize one or two fuel types for energy, the mitochondrial is incredibly versatile to be able to use all kinds of fuel. When you fast for longer periods (or are on a low-carb/ketogenic diet), your body begins to produce ketones, which are then used to cross the blood-brain barrier and fuel the brain in the absence of glucose. But that is not all. When you are in this fasted state of ketosis, the body will also increase the number of mitochondrial cells within your body, replacing non-mitochondrial cells with mitochondrial cells, allowing for more of your cells to be fueled by any fuel source.

Since the mitochondrial fuel ninety percent of the human body, by increasing the number of these cells, you can naturally increase your energy. Not only will your physical energy increase, but your mental functioning and energy will, as well. This is great news for many people who lose energy as they age.

Reduce Insulin Resistance

Insulin is perhaps the most well-known hormone, as the number of people diagnosed with diabetes only continues to rise. But insulin does not only affect people with diabetes but for everyone. This hormone, produced by the pancreas, is released after eating to allow the cells to absorb and utilize glucose as an energy source. But, often, our sensitivity to insulin decreases as we age or put on weight. The cells can become resistant to insulin, which leads to them being unable to absorb the glucose we have ingested. Over time, this causes a buildup of glucose in the bloodstream and, ultimately, diabetes if it is left untreated.

However, whether you have insulin resistance or already have been diagnosed with type II diabetes, you don't have to allow your condition to worsen. You can treat your insulin resistance directly at the source, and in the process, improve the absorption of glucose by your cells. Many people can lower the severity of their insulin resistance or diabetes, and some are even able to treat it completely.

Multiple controlled studies have found that intermittent fasting can both treat insulin resistance and lower blood glucose levels. Some studies have found that intermittent fasting can even be as effective, if not more effective, than dieting for lowering blood glucose levels.

Increase Neural Cells

It is important to take care of brain health as we age, especially as the levels of Alzheimer's disease, Parkinson's disease, and other neurodegenerative diseases are on the rise. But, one way that intermittent fasting can help guard against and treat all brain-related diseases is by increasing the production and repair of neural cells. This is important, as these diseases all cause these vital brain cells to become damaged or stunted overtime.

The result is that if you begin practicing intermittent fasting regularly now, you can reduce your risk of developing a neurological disease in the future. Or, if you already have one, you may be able to reduce symptoms or halt its progression. This is amazing news, as neurological diseases are incredibly hard to treat, even with modern medicine. Studies have specifically shown intermittent fasting to increase cell growth and repair in the cortex, hippocampus, basal forebrain, and nervous system. Along with the decreased risk of disease and disease progression, you can also expect to experience increased mental energy, better focus, improved memory, and a stabilized mood.

Lessen Oxidative Stress

Toxins cause oxidative stress. We can develop these toxins when we breathe in poor quality air, don't sleep well, eat poor quality food, apply damaging substances to our skin, and much more. We even develop this oxidative stress when our cells convert fuel to energy, meaning that even if we live in a clean environment, sleep perfectly, and only eat organic food, we would still develop oxidative stress, thereby causing damage to our cells. As our cells develop this damage from oxidative stress, we slowly lose our health and energy, producing an increased risk of disease.

However, studies have shown that intermittent fasting not only increases the rate our cells develop oxidative stress, but it also increases our body's natural antioxidants to fight against this damage directly.

Improve Mental Well-Being

Poor mental health is becoming more common than ever, with over forty-million Americans suffering from one form of mental illness or another, and many others struggling with short-term depression and anxiety. One of the most common causes of disability in middle-aged Americans (as well as those who are young) is chronic severe depression. Yet, a majority of these people never seek professional help.

While I urge you always to seek professional help for your mental health, you can also practice intermittent fasting. Studies have found that with short-term fasting, people can significantly improve their everyday mood, tranquility, alertness, and even the feeling of euphoria. Not only that but also the symptoms of severe depression can be improved with fasting.

Treat or Prevent Disease

While we cannot guarantee that intermittent fasting will prevent you from developing a disease or treat an infection you already have, many studies have proven that fasting can help. These studies have shown that fasting a person can menage their symptoms, possibly reverse the condition, and significantly reduce your likelihood of ever developing a disease. Now that we have looked at the general ways in which intermittent fasting can improve your health, let's have a look at some of the specific diseases and conditions you can expect short-term fasting to improve.

Less food consumption

One of the things you will notice over time is that you will begin to consume less food within your feasting window. Try to examine your food portions during your intermittent fast, and you'll see this clearly. Research shows that when fasting, you end up consuming 20% less food than the period before you began fasting. This is possibly due to the levels of the ghrelin hormone being normalized. Ghrelin is responsible for controlling appetite and triggering hunger, and in most of us, this hormone doesn't function efficiently. Due to our modern diet, a lot of our hormones are out of sync, which is why we feel hungry and eat all the time. Once your ghrelin starts working properly, you will feel less hungry.

It slows down the progression of cancer.

A study conducted on mice at the Duke University Medical Center in North Carolina showed that the caloric deficit resulting from intermittent fasting actually slowed down cancer in the mice.

Reduces Inflammation

Oxidative stress is one of the main reasons for inflammation in the body. Inflammation is the body's natural reaction to illness. However, excess inflammation is a painful condition and causes a host of diseases like arthritis. When the unstable molecules in the body, known as free radicals, react with other essential molecules like proteins and DNA, it causes inflammation. Intermittent fasting helps reduce inflammation and also offers protection against aging. Premature aging isn't desirable, now is it?

Heart's Health

Heart disease is the most significant killer in the world. Several risk factors increase the chance of heart disease. Intermittent fasting helps reduce risk factors like blood pressure, high cholesterol, inflammatory markers, blood sugar and blood triglycerides. When you can control these risk factors, you reduce the chance of suffering from cardiovascular disease. However, once again, a lot of research in this field is based on animal studies.

Cellular Repair

Autophagy is the process of waste removal in the body, and intermittent fasting helps to kick-start this process. The body breaks down and metabolizes broken, as well as dysfunctional, proteins. An increase in autophagy protects you from several degenerative diseases like cancer and Alzheimer's.

All these benefits help to increase your lifespan and help you lead a healthier life. Not only will you lose weight, but you can also improve your overall health just by following the intermittent fasting method.

Supports You in Healing Faster

When your cells have an easier time restoring themselves and your body is exposed to less stress, you have an easier time in healing faster. This means that any time you place a physical strain on your body, you can look forward to spending less time healing from that experience.

May Extend Your Lifespan

Intermittent fasting has shown in some studies that it may be able to extend your lifespan. Many people find themselves living shorter lives with poorer quality of life as a result of poor health. Disease and illness kill far more people each year than actual old age or natural causes do. Using the intermittent fasting diet may support you in preventing these illnesses and diseases so that you can live a longer, healthier, natural life.

Boosts Your Immune System

As a result of the many benefits that you gain from intermittent fasting, you also get to look forward to having an improved immune system. This is from the combination of reduced physical stress, increased cellular reparation abilities, weight loss, and other benefits that you gain from intermittent fasting.

Improved Sex Drive

Lower levels of production in both estrogen and testosterone may lead to a decreased sex drive. As such, it is not a psychological or physiological issue, but it is a hormonal matter. So, when you engage in intermittent fasting, your brain will regain its balance and begin to produce the right levels of all hormones.

So, in addition to improving your cognitive ability, restricting the production of cortisol, and boosting your mood through increased production of endorphins and dopamine, your body will also regulate the production of estrogen and testosterone which could potentially lead to a healthier sex drive.

Cellular Repair

Autophagy is the process of waste removal in the body, and intermittent fasting helps to kick-start this process. The body breaks down and metabolizes broken, as well as dysfunctional, proteins. An increase in autophagy protects you from several degenerative diseases like cancer and Alzheimer's.

All these benefits help to increase your lifespan and help you lead a healthier life. Not only will you lose weight, but you can also improve your overall health just by following the intermittent fasting method.

Chapter 4:
Pros and cons of intermittent fasting

There are pros and cons to every lifestyle. For instance, when you are eating a healthy and nutritious diet, you may lose weight and gain health but be unable to eat all your favorite foods in the amount you would like. On the other hand, when you eat junk food all the time you may enjoy yourself, but you will lose health and gain weight. In the same way, there are naturally both pros and cons to intermittent fasting, and by understanding what they are, you can better manage your lifestyle. Like all things, you will find that these pros and cons are most evened out when intermittent fasting is done in moderation. If a person only rarely practices fasting, then they will, in turn, only experience a few of the benefits. On the other hand, if they practice intermittent fasting overly enthusiastically and for longer periods than healthy, then they will experience more of the drawbacks.

Thankfully, with a balanced intermittent fasting schedule, you can find yourself experiencing many of the benefits and few, if any, of the drawbacks.

While some pros and cons of intermittent fasting are universal, others can be affected by gender and age. In this chapter, we will be exploring what pros and cons you individually may experience as a woman in or over her fifties.

Pros of Intermittent Fasting

Boost Weight Loss

Most people discover intermittent fasting either because they want to lose weight or gain health benefits. But, sometimes losing weight can accomplish both of those simultaneously, as a high body fat percentage can increase high blood pressure, cholesterol, and early mortality. Whether you are hoping to gain these health benefits by losing weight or wish to lose weight to feel more comfortable in your skin, you will love the way that intermittent fasting can boost your weight loss.

Balance Important Hormones

Thankfully, studies have found intermittent fasting can help balance a person's cortisol and melioration levels. It does this in a variety of ways. For instance, it can help to reduce cortisol by balancing and regulating blood sugar levels. By balancing cortisol, it sets off a chain reaction that improves the balance of other hormones, including melatonin. One simple change can benefit many hormones and systems within your body.

Improve Heart Health

As we age, we all must take even more care of our heart health. After all, heart disease is the number one killer of both men and women. While most often doctors educate men on the symptoms and warning signs of heart attacks, women are often forgotten, leading to increased risk of death. This means women must be extra vigilant, taking care of their heart health and educating themselves on the warning signs of heart attacks.

One crucial way to increase heart health is to watch your cholesterol. There is not a single type of cholesterol, but several. The two main types include LDL, which is known as the "bad" cholesterol, and HDL, known as the "good" cholesterol. While

LDL cholesterol will increase your risk of heart attack and heart disease, HDL cholesterol will protect your heart health and remove LDL cholesterol from your body.

Increase Mental Energy and Efficiency

We all need mental energy to get through the day. When our mind is sluggish, we are unable to think, accomplish anything, and sometimes we may be unable even to stay awake. We have all had troubles at times focusing on work, completing a math problem, remembering what we have read, and so on. This is all due to a lack of mental energy and efficiency. You may think that intermittent fasting would further reduce your mental state, as hunger makes focusing difficult, but the opposite is exact.

Reduce the Potential Risk of Developing Cancer

Of course, nobody can promise that any lifestyle choice will prevent you from developing cancer in the future. However, studies have found that intermittent fasting can potentially reduce your risk. Further studies are ongoing, but current research through animal studies have proven promising. For instance, it was found that rats with tumors survive longer when placed on fasting schedules than the control group.

Increase Longevity

Early studies on animals have found that by including intermittent fasting, an animal can experience an increased lifespan. These studies found that even if animals had a higher body fat percentage than the control group, by including intermittent fasting, they were able to increase their lifespan and longevity.

This makes sense, as intermittent fasting has many health benefits, and when all of these benefits are compounded together, it naturally results in a longer lifespan.

Lifestyle Ease

We all want improving health and weight, but it is important also to have an easier lifestyle. When it is difficult to gain health and weight, many of us end up failing, as life is already busy and difficult enough without adding added worry and tasks. If a person cook more, eat more frequently, and always worry about a diet, they are unlike to stick to it, as it is merely is unmaintainable.

It supports the secretion of the growth hormone.

It's present in kids more than in grown-ups, but it still helps a lot. The growth hormone decreases fat and improves the development of bone and muscles. It does this by turning glycogen to glucose into the bloodstream. This enables fat burn without the reduction of muscles. When you sleep and exercise enough, the growth hormone is also boosted.

It enables you to avoid heart illnesses.

Both blood glucose control and fat loss are done by IF improve heart health. The likelihood of getting coronary artery heart illness can also be reduced.

Intermittent fasting is very versatile and can fit in any schedule.

It is not as challenging as certain diets that unnecessarily trigger a huge disturbance in your life. There is no particular time to perform the IF. They can be blended as you think it is appropriate for your timetable. You are not boxed into any regiment that you cannot retain easily. Intermittent rapidity adapts to life's unpredictability. This can also be practiced everywhere in the globe as there is no special gear you need so as to do it; it only restricts your feeding and is therefore much easier and more practical than many diets. It's completely all right, even if you have to halt fasting for a while. In a matter of minutes, you can begin fasting again.

It accepts all food

Organic foods have more nutrients than processed foods. These organic products are unfortunately quite costly, so purchasing them will diminish your pockets every day. In fact, they can be almost 10 times more expensive than processed products. It is obviously easier to afford processed products as they are cheap. No matter the effectiveness of a diet, if you can't afford it, it cannot help you at all. Fasting is in the first position of cost-effectiveness since it is completely free. You don't have to purchase any meals, so it costs you no cash. There's no reason for you to purchase costly meals or supplements or any drug that makes it cheap for all.

Simple to practice

Intermediate fasting is easy to do and doesn't have any complicated scheduling, it is quite direct. This causes it to be simpler to pursue and more efficient than many diets.

Opens up your mind

It enables you to regulate your mental procedures as IF opens up your body. You are used to responding to your body's urges because you consume whenever you feel slightly hungry. You are released from the control of your body as a result of practicing IF.

Corrects insulin resistance

This is the simplest and easiest route to reduce insulin resistance and insulin levels. It has a highly effective impact. It works better than a rigid low carb diet.

Improves your metabolism

Intermittent fasting enhances your metabolism by considerably reducing the number of calories you eat in one day. During the feeding time you have, it is almost possible to eat the suggested daily calorific requirements. This causes modifications in the body and fat burning. It also helps you to burn fat, even if you eat the normal calories as your system requires, as it will make you burn fat for power instead of carbs.

Cons of Intermittent Fasting

Getting Started Takes an Adjustment

Any lifestyle change takes an adjustment, and it can take months for something to become a habit. Naturally, intermittent fasting is quite an adjustment for people who are used to grazing on food throughout the day. This means that if you push yourself to go into an advanced version of intermittent fasting when you first begin, you can become overwhelmed. But if you start slowly and allow your body to adjust in its own time, you will find it happens much more naturally and becomes easy to stick to.

Potential to Overeat

While intermittent fasting should naturally reduce caloric intake, if a person pushes themselves to fast when they are overly hungry, it might lead to overeating during their eating window. This is because the person feels hungry for so long when fasting when they can finally eat their body believes it must make up for the calories it missed. The result is that the person either hits a weight loss plateau or even experience increased weight.

Possible Leptin Imbalance

The hormone leptin is important as it signals to your body that you are full have no longer need to eat. But when a person practices intermittent fasting, it may temporarily disrupt this hormone's production. However, this is usually only a short-term problem, and once a person's body adjusts to their fasting and eating windows, their leptin will balance itself out.Typically, a leptin imbalance is only a real problem when a person dives head-first into intermittent fasting and attempt to practice advanced level fasting when they are still only a beginner.

Not Everyone Can Practice Intermittent Fasting

Intermittent fasting is a beautiful and healthy lifestyle for the general population. After all, the human body is designed for practice periods of fasting naturally. However, not every person can practice fasting. Some people, due to chronic illness, may be unable to participate. Ultimately, you must ask your doctor if you are healthy enough to practice short-term fasting.

It can trigger the re-feeding syndrome

This is a hazardous and fatal disorder that can happen if you suffer from malnutrition. It is when electrolyte and liquid imbalances occur when malnourished individuals have been hospitalized for a long time and eat again after a long time. The chance of acquiring re-feeding syndrome increases when bodily weight is very small and not eating for more than ten days.

Having low energy.

Although after a while starvation passes, life isn't predictable. You can take part in a tiresome activity that makes you hungry and ultimately unproductive until the hunger goes or you eat. You may have been used to eating a bunch of snacks during the day and quit instantly due to fasting, which may cause a few side-effects. These side effects involve headaches, bad temper, and lack of power, constipation and low levels of concentration. It may also decrease your motivation. This sort of fasting can have an adverse fitness effect if you have a health condition. It is not suitable for all. For example, hypoglycemic people require glucose all day, so they can't profit from fasting.

Interfere with the social side of eating

Eating from ancient times was a significant social event. Special times, festivities, milestone accomplishment and other activities require meal sharing with your friends. IF can mess with your personal life when you change your routine which may not correspond to the regular eating schedule. During occasions where everyone eats and eats, you may stand out as the one who does not want to participate. Many activities including dinner meetings, family meals, and romantic meals are missed among many others.

Reproductive complications in some women

If the fasting is carried out in a fashion that mainly restricts carbs and protein, it can trigger fertility problems in females, lead to electrolyte defects and trigger nutritional deficits. There are also long-term adverse health effects. Intermediate fasting is linked to menstrual, premature menopause and health problems. Research indicates that ovary size can be reduced, thus influencing reproduction, in addition to decreasing bodily volume.

Digestive complications

It can lead to problems linked to digestion. When food is eaten too rapidly, a large meal may cause digestive problems. People who tend to have larger dishes during the feeding period, require to digest them for a longer period of time. It increases the pressure on your digestive system, triggering indigestion and bloating. This will have a stronger impact on people with weak guts.

Weight regains

Intermittent acceleration reduces the body's reliance on carbohydrates for fuel and decreases fat dependency for power. There is an improvement in the decomposition of stored fats. The body undergoes physiological changes as a reaction to a drastic decrease in the body's power consumption. Simply put, this implies that you may not be able to keep your weight or even gain more weight despite extreme dietary restrictions.

Having seen the strengths and downsides of this fasting protocol, it is evident that the amount and weight of each benefit is more advantageous than the downsides. Intermittent fasting will greatly improve the quality and the quantity of your life without a doubt.

Chapter 5:
Enhancing intermittent fasting for you

Intermittent fasting is much easier than people first believe, as you pair your fasting periods with feasting periods full of nutritious and satisfying food. Therefore, you stay full during your fasting period, much unlike the meal skipping that most people experience. As long as you start slowly and allow your body to adjust naturally, it should be a simple process. Although, if you do struggle, you should find that after the first five days, things become easier, as after this period, your body will begin to adjust, and fasting will become routine. In this chapter, we will go over some tips and tricks that can make your intermittent fasting journey easier, helping you to gain success, lose weight, and achieve better health.

Research, Research, Research

It's easy to want to jump right into intermittent fasting once you learn of the benefits it has to offer and humanity's history of naturally including fasting in daily life. But if you jump head-first into a new lifestyle without fully understanding it, you are likely to make mistakes that you will later regret.

Understand Your Motivation

Making a lifestyle change when only half understanding your motivation is a setting yourself up to quit halfway through. Any lifestyle change takes effort, and if we only have vague ideas of "I want to be healthier" or "I want to weigh less," we can quickly become defeated at the first sign of hurdles. Instead, sit down and write out a list of attainable goals you hope to succeed with. For instance, what aspects of your health do you want to improve? Do you want to lower your cholesterol? Improve your blood pressure? Manage your blood sugar? Reduce daily fatigue? Reduce insomnia to get two more hours of sleep a night? If you want to lose weight, set yourself both short-term and long-term goals. For instance, in the short-term, you can try to lose ten pounds, but maybe long-term, you want to lose fifty.

By having these goals, you will be motivated to overcome the hurdles that come your way, gaining success, and enjoying a better lifestyle.

Slow and Steady Wins the Race

When you are excited about succeeding, losing weight, and gaining health, then it is easy to want to rush into intermittent fasting. After you are armed with all the knowledge you need to succeed, you might want to start right off with a 16/8 or even a 20/4 fast. But this is only setting yourself up for failure, just like the hare in the fable "The Tortoise and the Hare." Instead of seeking the fastest way to your goal, find the most successful approach. What does this mean? Don't jump into the more difficult fasting periods. Rather, start with a 12/12 fast or skipping a meal when you aren't hungry. Just be sure that when you do eat that you eat healthy and nutritious food! You can also start by cutting out snacks and training both your mind and body to not eat between mealtimes. After you adjust to these smaller changes, you can slightly increase your fasting window every few days until you reach your desired fasting length.

Drink Plenty of Water

The importance of staying hydrated cannot be overstated. The truth is that most Americans do not drink their recommended daily intake, which can lead to headaches, migraines, fatigue, stress, false hunger pangs, and more. In fact, by the time you are feeling thirsty, you already are slightly dehydrated. Don't forget to drink your daily intake of water, which is half of your body's weight in pounds in ounces. This means that if you weigh one-hundred and fifty pounds, you should be drinking seventy-five fluid ounces of water, at least, daily.

When you are dehydrated, you can experience false hunger pangs, making you believe that you need to eat when you don't. If you find yourself feeling hungry during your fasting window, before ending your fast early and eating a snack, instead try drinking a glass of water. If you have trouble remembering to drink water, then keep a reusable water bottle at hand at all times and try using a water tracking smartphone app.

Avoid Temptation

While we may not always avoid being around our favorite tempting foods when possible, don't put yourself in a situation to give in to your cravings. For instance, if you know you have a habit of giving in and eating specific junk foods, try not to keep them at home.

But, avoiding temptation is not always about avoiding your favorite foods, but rather timing when you eat them. For instance, if you have a plan to go out to coffee or for drinks with friends, then don't plan your fast during this time. Instead, work your fast around your schedule so that you can enjoy getting food and drinks with friends without impeding your fasting schedule or weight loss. You can still fully enjoy yourself and experience the benefits of intermittent fasting.

You might also consider tailoring where you go out with friends based on the menu. If you are trying to lower your blood sugar, then instead of going out for ice cream, it would be better for your health to find a healthier alternative until your fasting schedule improves your health. Instead of ice cream, you might choose to go out for coffee or get a slightly healthier dessert option, even.

Enjoy the Caffeine Boost

If you have high blood pressure, you should watch the caffeine, but if you have normal or low blood pressure, you can generally feel free to enjoy a caffeine boost you help you through your fast. Of course, like all medical decisions, you should ask your doctor about your personalized caffeine intake recommendation.

You will find that caffeine can be especially helpful when you are first adjusting to a fasting lifestyle, as it can reduce appetite, helping you to feel more satisfied between meals. Not only that, but it also will provide you with a nice energy boost.

Just remember not to add anything with calories to your coffee during a fasting window, meaning no sugar, cream, or milk. Save these ingredients for your eating windows, instead. If you dislike black coffee or tea, you can add sugar-free natural stevia sweetener during a fasting window. You can also use sugar-free gum to help reduce cravings during the initial adjustment period.

Stay Busy

It's easy to think that you don't want to stress while busy, and while you may want to avoid changing lifestyles during stressful periods, it is best to take up intermittent fasting when you are working. After all, many people will snack out of boredom, or at the very least, are more likely to notice hunger pangs when they have nothing but time on their hands. On the other hand, if you stay busy with work, chores, or hobbies, you will be able to get through the fasting period seemingly more quickly, with fewer noticeable hunger pangs or temptations to snack.

Remember, a watched pot never boils, and time seems to move most slowly when you are watching the clock. So, if you fast when you are too busy to notice the hours pass by, you will find that before you know it, your fasting window ends, and you can enjoy your next meal. This doesn't mean you need to take up intermittent fasting when your job is keeping you busy, but at the very least, try to find tasks you can delve into at home to pass the time.

Liberally Season Your Food

Surprisingly to many people, by piling on the seasonings during meals in the way of spices, herbs, and vinegar, you can wake up your taste buds, thereby feeling satisfied and full for longer periods. These ingredients also contain very few calories, meaning you can add them liberally to your dishes without adverse effects on your weight.

In Western countries, many people under season their dishes, as you can tell when you compare typical American or British dishes to those from Asia, the Middle East, and other countries throughout the world. Instead of merely cooking fish or chicken with a little salt and pepper, try using a recipe that uses a handful of different spices, herbs, and vinegar so that you can enjoy a genuinely flavorful dish. Not only will these dishes help keep you satisfied, but you will also find that they taste better and are more enjoyable.

Prioritize High-Quality and Consistent Sleep

Sleep is a vital part of health and well-being, and that includes our health while practicing intermittent fasting. Not only that but by scheduling your fasting schedule to overlap with your sleeping schedule, you can accomplish a longer fasting window without hunger. Without trying, we all already fast overnight between dinner and breakfast, so with a little knowledge of intermittent fasting, you can make better use of this time.

If you are going to be having a particularly long overnight fast, it can help to go to sleep early so that you do not become tempted to get a midnight snack. Although, keep in mind that some people find that an overly large dinner can interrupt their quality of sleep, so find what best works for both your sleep and your fasting schedule. When leading a busy life, or distracted by a good book or TV show, it is easy to neglect sleep. But you mustn't do this, as when you do not sleep properly, it will alter your hormonal balance. As you become sleep deprived, the hormone cortisol will increase, which not only increases stress and impedes sleep but also increases hunger and weight gain. Leptin and ghrelin will also become unbalanced, further increasing hunger and overeating, thereby blocking your progress.

Only by prioritizing consistent and high-quality sleep, you can significantly increase your success in fasting, but also improve your overall health and weight.

Track Your Progress

While you shouldn't obsess or hyper-focus on your fasting schedule and results, as this can make people overly stressed and self-conscious, it is important to at least track the basics of your progress. This is because it can sometimes feel like we are not making any progress as the scale is not moving, and then you realize you are actually down two jean sizes. The range is not always accurate; what is more important is how fat is positioned on your body.

Therefore, don't only weigh yourself, but also measure your stomach, hips, waist, bust, chest, upper arms, forearms, thighs, and calves. You don't have to worry about tracking these measurements or your weight daily, but at least monitor them once every week or every two weeks. And remember, when you do check your weight and measurements, write it down to keep a record!

By tracking your progress, not only will you be able to recognize your achievement better as you are making it, but you will also come to understand your body and its patterns better.

You can track your progress in a small notebook, journal, yearly planner, or there are even several of helpful smartphone apps created for this purpose.

Avoid Fasting When Stressed

We all have times in our life when everything seems to be going wrong. Perhaps a loved one is in the hospital, something happened to a beloved family pet, or you are going through a breakup. Generally, these are not good times to begin a new lifestyle. Sure, sometimes you may not be able to avoid it if you need to improve your heart health or blood sugar, but if you can help it, try to begin intermittent fasting when life does feel like a burden. If you do choose to practice fasting during these times, offer yourself kindness and compassion. You can practice shorter fasting windows rather than going for more advanced fasting windows. Allow yourself to have a comforting treat from time to time. If you mess up, forgive yourself.

When making a lifestyle change, you must practice self-kindness if you hope to succeed.

Chapter 6:
Weight loss and healthy living

There are so many different reasons why we all gain weight. Some people think everyone that is obese sits around eating junk all day. Sure, maybe some do this, but in general, there is usually an underlying health reason that someone might have struggles when trying to lose weight and reduce their overall weight gain.

Cause of Weight Gain

If you are eating foods that are high in salt, then this can cause your body to hold onto a lot of weight through excess water. This will usually show itself in visual places, such as your chin/chest, your feet, or your hands. When you first start on a healthy diet, you might drop 20 pounds in as quick as a month.

This is because your body is letting go of that water. Then, as weight loss progresses, it becomes a lot slower, because you're not holding onto that water. This can be very discouraging for some. They might start a drastic diet, losing five pounds in just a week. Then, however, they might gain back three pounds the next week, and think that the diet doesn't work, quitting, and moving on. Always remember water retention in the struggle for weight loss.

Our bodies can sometimes resist our attempt at weight loss as well. If you are participating in extreme diets like only drinking lemon water for a week, but then go back to eating unhealthily next week, you're confusing your body. It will resist that diet in the first place in order to better deal with the fluctuations you're seeing. This is why you might feel like you gain weight quickly, or why if you lose weight, it doesn't always stay off.

Another cause of weight gain can be not eating right, along with exercising. You might be an active person, or know an active person, who frequently works out or participate in sports. Despite their dedication, they're still overweight. The biggest reason for this is unhealthy eating. Some people can get away with eating unhealthily and exercising and still having a low body weight and fit physique. However, for the most part, it's crucial that we also focus on healthier diets in addition to whichever workout we choose to add.

Alternatively, some people think they don't have to exercise at all, and the weight will just come off. In the beginning, this is true. If you don't work out and don't eat healthily, but then start to eat healthy food, you will lose some weight. You will eventually plateau, however, especially after your stomach and metabolism adjust. Not everyone has to dedicate an hour a day at the gym. However, light and frequent cardio, such as a walk every other day or 20 minutes on the treadmill a day are still very important if you want to lose weight continually.

There are many sneaky foods that will get into our diets and cause us to hang onto unwanted weight as well. The biggest hidden food is sugar. This will often be found in highly processed foods. Some things might market themselves as organic, making you think "healthy." They might also show pictures of fruits and veggies, stating things like "contains two whole apples, one berry, one banana, etc." What they won't put on the front, however, is that they also contain %30 of your daily recommended sugar!

Things like yogurt, deli meats, frozen veggies, and other processed foods that are seemingly harmless might very well contain high levels of sodium, which will cause water retention, and high levels of sugar, which can imbalance your hormones and cause a higher amount of fat to be stored throughout your body.

Dehydration is another culprit of obesity. Water needs to be consumed in certain amounts depending on your body weight, regardless if you drink other beverages. Some people might think that they had some coffee, juice, tea, or even a soda, and think this counts towards their hydration level. However, some of these will contain things that can even dehydrate you further, so it's crucial that you never deprive yourself an excessive amount of water.

One of the biggest reasons that we might struggle with obesity and the overall ability to lose weight is because of the mentality around dieting. To lose weight doesn't mean to give up food for a month, and then the pounds come off and stay off. There's no pill, shake, or surgery that will help you stay in shape. These things will remove fat, but they won't keep them off and can end up causing you to gain more weight later on because of the intense fluctuation in debt we're giving our bodies. If you really want to lose weight and fight obesity, then we need to work with our body's natural fat-burning properties.

A Healthy and Balanced Diet

Fasting is a great way to lose weight. However, if you are eating unhealthy during the periods that you do eat, then fasting isn't going to end up doing you any good. Your body will eventually balance out.

You should be eating a balanced diet even if you read this book through and then decide fasting isn't for you. The combination of both, along with exercise, is going to be your secret to melting your body fat, however. Throughout this chapter, we are going to take a look at some of the best ways that you can burn your body fat through a healthy and balanced diet.

The biggest mistake dieters will make is by purchasing and focusing only on "diet," "organic," "natural," and other types of foods that are only labeled for being healthy. Don't be misguided by some fancy wording, especially blank statements like "part of a complete meal." Any meal could be complete! "Part of a healthy meal," is something that is actually saying something of value.

Start by cutting out as many processed foods as possible. We'll all have those pizza cravings after a night out at the bar or want to indulge in a sugary coffee with our breakfasts. However, you should be putting an emphasis on having these things as treats. If you have them every once in a while, your body will be able to process them easier, meaning it's not like you'll gain two pounds from having one slice of cake. However, if you have a slice of cake every day, you will start to gain weight again. Don't think you have to cut them out of your life altogether – this is the kind of all or nothing thinking that can send us into a panic and want to binge.

Of course, you might struggle with your control over food and find it difficult to have "just a few" of certain kinds of sweets. Still, make it a priority to reduce the number of junk food items you add in regularly.

Choose whole wheat over white carbs, such as whole-wheat bread versus white bread, whole-grain pasta over white pasta, and so on. Pick lean meat like chicken and fish over heavier red meat like bacon and steak.

Pick fresh fruits and veggies over canned, and make sure if you do buy frozen that there are no additives. Always check your labels and make sure the sugar, salt, and fat content are lower than other vitamin and mineral counts that might be labeled.

Don't think you can't snack either. Smaller meals combined with healthier snacks throughout the day is always a better choice than just three huge meals.

Regulating Your Metabolism

The reason that some people will include cheat days in their diet is first to alleviate some of the pressures of dieting and give into their biggest cravings. It's also helpful in keeping your metabolism on its toes. Combined with fasting, this will help keep your metabolism active and regulated rather than sticking to one diet, and one kind of food, all the time.

Your metabolism is based on weight, age, and sex. The younger you are, the bigger you are, and the more muscles you have, the faster you burn food. Men typically have more muscles than women (think hips/breasts/and other fatty areas on women), which is why it might be easier for a husband to lose weight after giving up soda, while his wife struggles to lose a pound even though she eats nothing but salad. The combination of a balanced diet with fasting will help to keep your metabolism regulated.

How to Use Fasting for Weight Loss

All of this means that adding fasting to whatever else you are doing will help you to lose weight. The more of these healthy habits you can add into your life, such as focusing on balanced meals and exercise, the better results you will see.

Fasting can burn fat, detoxify your body, and help build self-control. All of this can lead to a healthier lifestyle you've been looking for.

Chapter 7:
Breakfast

Zucchini Omelet

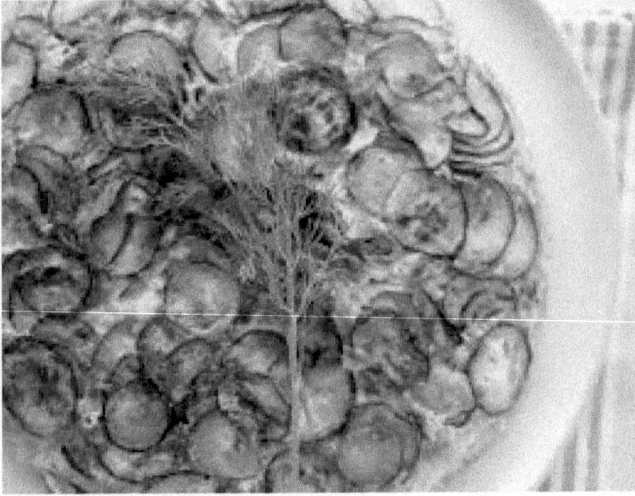

Preparation time: 4 minutes

Cooking time: 3 hours and 30 minutes

Servings: 6

Ingredients:

1½ cups red onion, chopped

1 tablespoon olive oil

2 garlic cloves, minced

2 teaspoons fresh basil, chopped

6 eggs, whisked

A pinch of sea salt and black pepper

8 cups zucchini, sliced

6 ounces fresh tomatoes, peeled, crushed

Directions

In a bowl, mix all the ingredients except the oil and the basil.

Grease the slow cooker with the oil, spread the omelet mix in the bowl, cover and cook on low for 3 hours and 30 minutes.

Divide the omelet between plates, sprinkle the basil on top and serve for breakfast.

Nutritional info: Calories: 120, Fat: 18g, Protein: 15g, Carbs: 1.8g

Chili Omelet

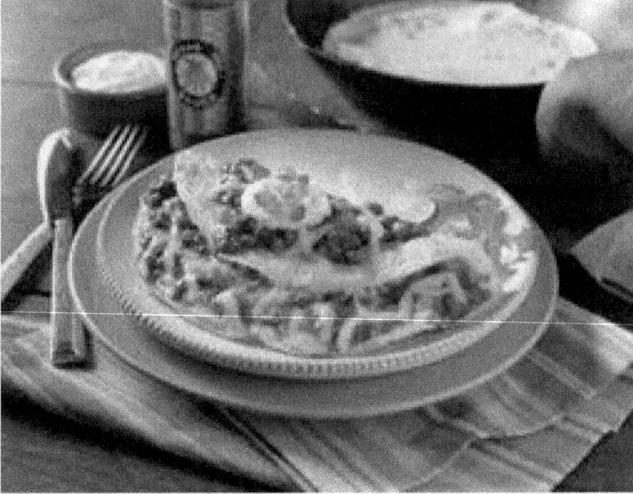

Preparation time: 5 minutes

Cooking time: 3 hours and 30 minutes

Servings: 4

Ingredients:

2 garlic cloves, minced

1 tablespoon olive oil

1 red bell pepper, chopped

1 small yellow onion, chopped

1 teaspoon chili powder

2 tablespoons tomato puree

½ teaspoon sweet paprika

A pinch of salt and black pepper

1 tablespoon parsley, chopped

4 eggs, whisked

Directions

In a bowl, mix all the ingredients except the oil and the parsley and whisk them well.

Grease the slow cooker with the oil, add the egg mixture, cover and cook on low for 3 hours and 30 minutes.

Divide the omelet between plates, sprinkle the parsley on top and serve for breakfast.

Nutritional info: Calories: 100, Fat: 10g, Protein: 15g, Carbs: 1.8g

Basil and Cherry Tomato Breakfast

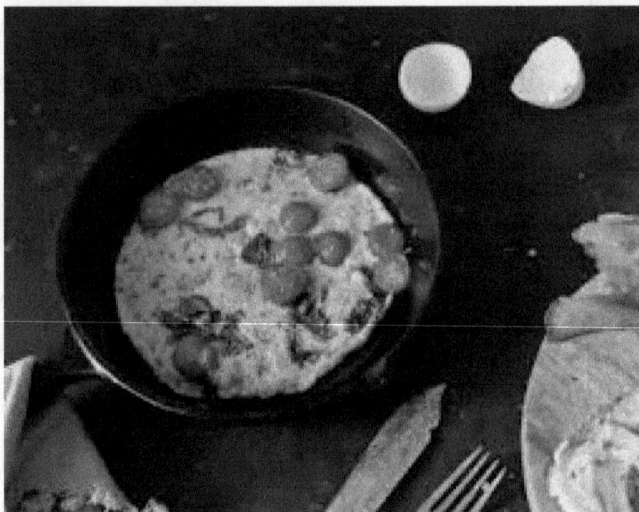

Preparation time: 4 minutes

Cooking time: 4 hours

Servings: 4

Ingredients:

1 tablespoon olive oil

2 yellow onions, chopped

2 pounds cherry tomatoes, halved

3 tablespoons tomato puree

2 garlic cloves, minced

A pinch of sea salt and black pepper

1 bunch basil, chopped

Directions

Grease the slow cooker with the oil, add all the ingredients, cover and cook on high for 4 hours.

Stir the mixture, divide it into bowls and serve for breakfast.

Nutritional info: Calories: 90, Fat: 1g, Protein: 1g, Carbs: 1.8g

Carrot Breakfast Salad

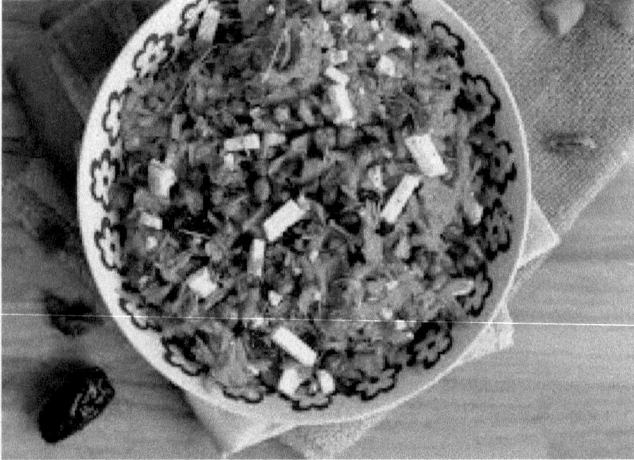

Preparation time: 5 minutes

Cooking time: 4 ho urs

Servings: 4

Ingredients:

2 tablespoons olive oil

2 pounds baby carrots, peeled and halved

3 garlic cloves, minced

2 yellow onions, chopped

½ cup vegetable stock

1/3 cup tomatoes, crushed

A pinch of salt and black pepper

Directions

In your slow cooker, combine all the ingredients, cover and cook on high for 4 hours.

Divide into bowls and serve for breakfast.

Nutritional info: Calories: 50, Fat: 10g, Protein: 10g, Carbs: 1.8g

Garlic Zucchini Mix

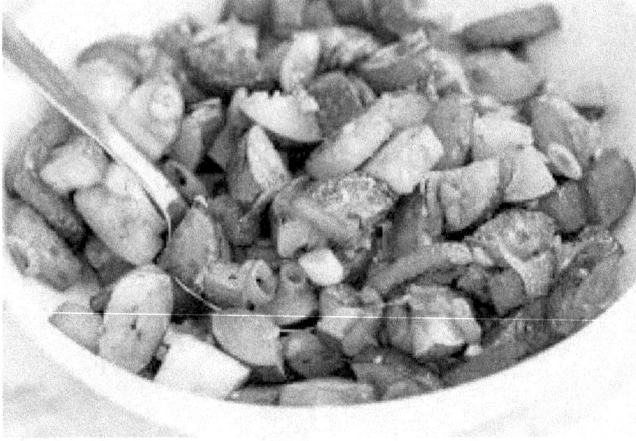

Preparation time: 5 minutes

Cooking time: 6 hours

Servings: 6

Ingredients:

4 cups zucchinis, sliced

2 tablespoons olive oil

1 teaspoon Italian seasoning

A pinch of salt and black pepper

1 teaspoon garlic powder

Directions

In your slow cooker, mix all the ingredients, cover and cook on Low for 6 hours.

Divide into bowls and serve for breakfast.

Nutritional info: Calories: 60, Fat: 0.7g, Protein: 1.5g, Carbs: 1.8g

Crustless Broccoli Sun-dried Tomato Quiche

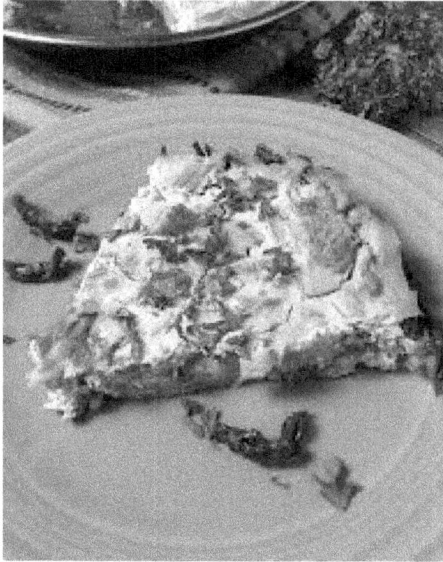

Preparation time: 4 minutes

Cooking time: 3 hours and 30 mi nutes

Servings: 6

Ingredients:

12.3-ounce box extra-firm tofu drained and dried

1 ½ cup broccoli, chopped

2 teaspoons yellow mustard

1 tablespoon tahini

1 tablespoon cornstarch

¼ cup old fashioned oats

½ teaspoon turmeric

3-4 dashes Tabasco sauce

½-1 teaspoon salt

½ cup artichoke hearts, chopped

2/3 cup tomatoes, sun-dried, soaked in hot water

1/8 cup vegetable broth

Directions

Preheat your oven to 375 degrees Fahrenheit.

Prepare a 9" pie plate or springform pan with parchment paper or cooking spray.

Put all of the leeks and broccoli on a cookie sheet and drizzle with vegetable broth, salt, and pepper. Bake for about 20-30 min.

In the meantime, add the tofu, garlic, nutritional yeast, lemon juice, mustard, tahini, cornstarch, oats, turmeric, salt, and a few dashes of Tabasco in a food processor. When the mixture is smooth, taste for heat and add more Tabasco as needed.

Place cooked vegetables with artichoke hearts and tomatoes in a large bowl. With a spatula, scrape in tofu mixture from the processor. Mix carefully, so all of the vegetables are well distributed. If the mixture seems too dry, add a little vegetable broth or water.

Add mixture to pie plate muffin tins, or springform pan and spread evenly.

Bake for about 35 min. or until lightly browned.

Cool before serving. It is delicious, both warm and chilled!

Nutritional info: Calories: 150, Fat: 18g, Protein: 15g, Carbs: 1.8g

Chocolate Pancakes

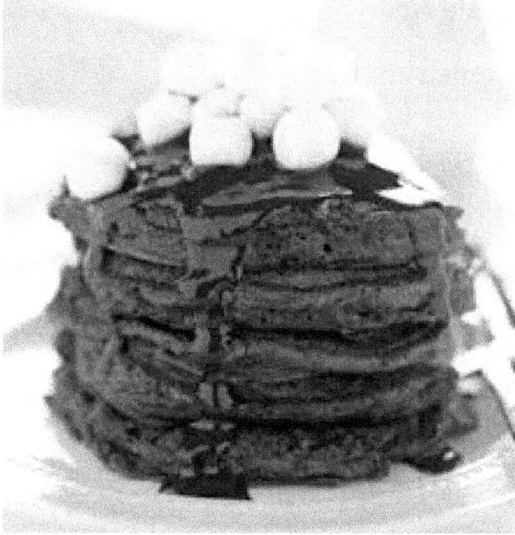

Preparation time: 5 minutes

Cooking time: 80 min utes

Servings: 6

Ingredients:

1 ¼ cup gluten-free flour of choice

1 tablespoon ground flaxseed

1 tablespoon baking powder

3 tablespoons nutritional yeast

2 tablespoons unsweetened cocoa powder

¼ teaspoon of sea salt

1 cup unsweetened, unflavored almond milk

1 tablespoon vegan mini chocolate chips (optional)

1 teaspoon vanilla extract

¼ teaspoon stevia powder or 1 tablespoon pure maple syrup

1 tablespoon apple cider vinegar

¼ cup unsweetened applesauce.

Directions

Get a medium bowl and mix all the dry ingredients (flour, baking powder, flaxseed, cocoa powder, yeast, salt, and optional chocolate chips). Whisk until evenly combined.

In a separate small bowl, combine wet ingredients except for the applesauce (almond milk, vanilla extract, apple cider vinegar, maple syrup, or stevia powder).

Add wet ingredient mixture and applesauce to the dry ingredients and mix by hand until ingredients are just combined.

The batter should sit for 10 minutes. It will rise and thicken, possibly doubling in size.

Heat an electric griddle or nonstick skillet to medium heat and spray with a small amount of nonstick spray, if desired. Scoop batter into 3-inch rounds. Much like traditional pancakes, bubbles will start to appear. When bubbles start to burst, flip pancakes and cook for 1-2 minutes. Yields 12 pancakes.

Nutritional info: Calories: 150, Fat: 18g, Protein: 15g, Carbs: 1.8g

Breakfast Scramble

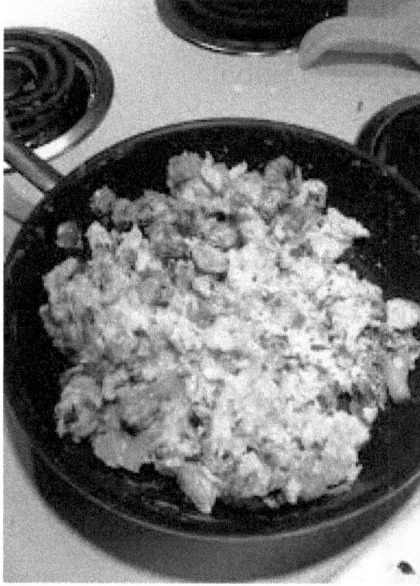

Preparation time: 5 minutes

Cooking time: 60 min utes

Servings: 7

Ingredients:

1 large head cauliflower, cut up

1 seeded, diced green bell pepper

1 seeded, diced red bell pepper

2 cups sliced mushrooms (approximately 8 oz whole mushrooms)

1 peeled, diced red onion

3 peeled, minced cloves of garlic

Sea salt

1 ½ teaspoons turmeric

1–2 tablespoons of low-sodium soy sauce

¼ cup nutritional yeast (optional)

½ teaspoon black pepper

Directions

1. Sauté green and red peppers, mushrooms, and onion in a medium saucepan or skillet over medium-high heat until onion is translucent (should be 7–8 min). Add an occasional tablespoon or two of water to the pan to prevent vegetables from sticking.

2. Add cauliflower and cook until florets are tenders. It should be 5 to 6 minutes.

3. Add, pepper, garlic, soy sauce, turmeric, and yeast (if using) to the pan and cook for about 5 minutes.

Nutritional info: Calories: 180, Fat: 18g, Protein: 15g, Carbs: 1.8g

Oatmeal

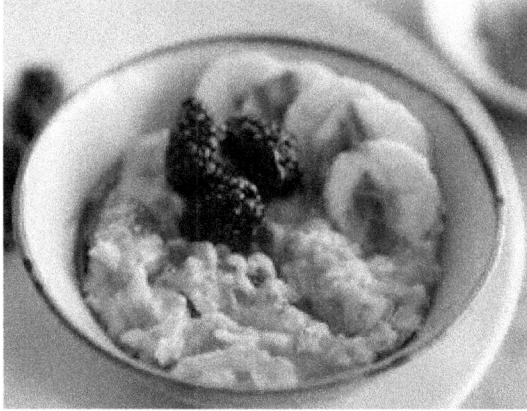

Preparation time: 5 minutes

Cooking time: 30 minutes

Servings: 4 Serves

Ingredients:

Almond milk, unsweetened, one cup

Flaxseed, whole, one tablespoon

Sunflower seeds, one tablespoon

Chia seeds, one tablespoon

Salt, one half teaspoon

Directions

Dump all of the ingredients together into a small pan and bring the mixture to a boil in a saucepan over medium heat. When it comes to a boil, reduce the heat and allow the mix to simmer gently for two to three minutes until the mix is the desired thickness. Drop a pat of butter on the top and enjoy.

Nutrition per serving:

Calories 621, 9 grams net carbs, 62 grams fat, 10 grams protein

Coconut Cream with Berries

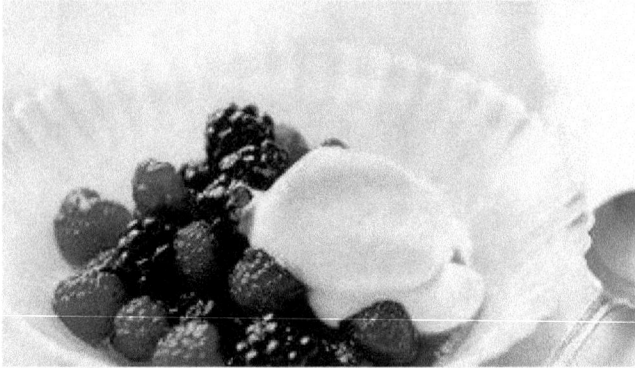

Preparation time: 5 minutes

Cooking time: 30 minutes

Servings: 4 Serves

Ingredients:

Coconut cream, one ha lf cup

Vanilla extract, one teaspoon

Strawberries, fresh, two ounces

Directions

Mix the ingredients together well by using a hand mixer or an immersion mixer if one is available. An added teaspoon of coconut oil will increase the amount of fat in this dish.

Nutrition per serving:

Calories 415, 9 grams net carbs, 42 grams fat, 5 grams protein

Seafood Omelet

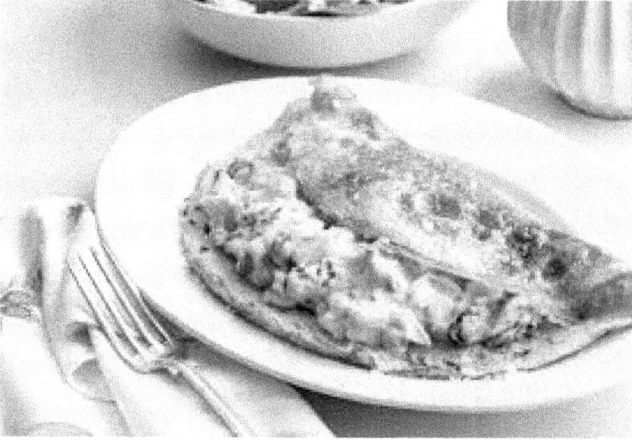

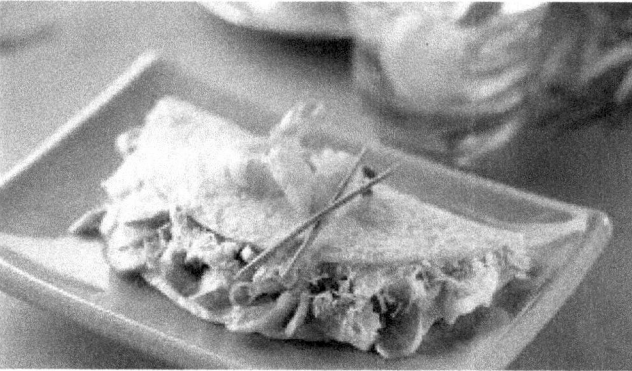

Preparation time: 5 minutes

Cooking time: 30 minutes

Serves two

Ingredients:

Shrimp, cooked, five ounces

Eggs, six

Butter, two tablespoons

Olive oil, two tablespoons

Chives, fresh or dried, one tablespoon

Mayonnaise, one half cup

Cumin, ground, one half teaspoon

Thyme, one quarter teaspoon

Garlic, two cloves minced

Red chili pepper, one diced

Salt, one half teaspoon

White pepper, one teaspoon

Directions

Toss the shrimp with the olive oil until it is completely covered and fry it gently with the cumin, garlic, salt, chili pepper, and pepper for five minutes. While the shrimp mix cools beat the eggs and pours them into the skillet. Let the eggs sit undisturbed while they cook until the edges begin to brown and the center has mostly set firm. Then add the chives and the mayonnaise to the shrimp mixture. Pour the shrimp mixture onto the egg that is frying in the skillet and fold the omelet in half, frying for an additional three minutes on each side.

Nutrition per serving:

Calories 872, 4 grams net carbs, 83 grams fat, 27 grams protein

Spinach and Pork with Fried Eggs

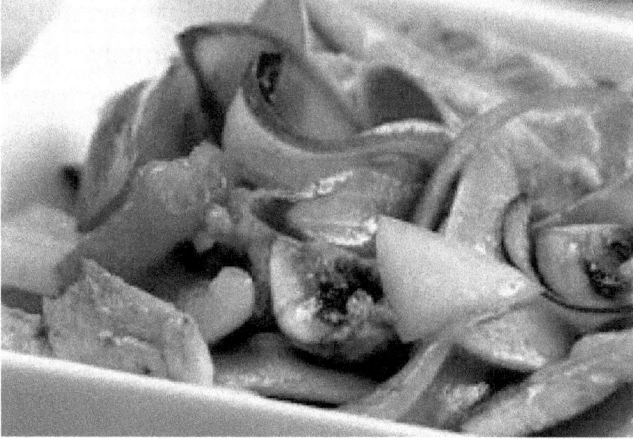

Preparation time: 5 minutes

Cooking time: 30 minutes

Serves two

Ingredients:

Spinach, baby, two cups

Pork loin, smoked, six ounces cut into chunks

Eggs, four

Salt, one half teaspoon

Black pepper, one teaspoon

Walnuts, chopped, one quarter cup

Cranberries, one quarter cup frozen

Butter, three tablespoons

Directions

Wash, dry, and chop the baby spinach. Fry the spinach in the butter for five minutes stirring continuously. Remove the spinach from the pan and let it drain on a paper towel. Fry the chunks of pork loin in the same skillet for five minutes. Remove the pork from the skillet and then put the cooked baby spinach back in, adding the nuts and cranberries. Stir constantly while this is cooking for five minutes. Pour the mix into a bowl. Fry the eggs and place two on each plate with half of the spinach mixture. Serve with the chunks of fried pork loin.

Nutrition per serving:

Calories 1033, 8 grams net carbs, 99 grams fat, 26 grams protein

Smoked Salmon Sandwich

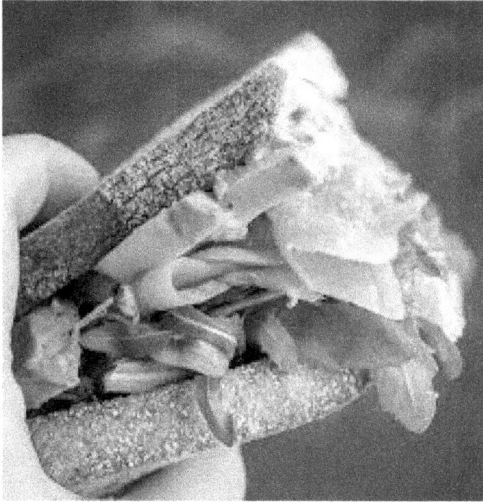

Preparation time: 5 minutes

Cooking time: 30 minutes

Serves two

Ingredients:

TOPPING

Eggs, four

Chives, fresh, chop, one tablespoon

Smoked salmon, three ounces

Heavy whipping cream, two tablespoons

Salt, one half teaspoon

White pepper, one half teaspoon

Kale, one-ounce chop fine

Butter, two tablespoons

Chili powder, one quarter teaspoon

Olive oil, two tablespoons

SPICY PUMPKIN BREAD

Lard, one tablespoon

Pumpkin puree, fourteen ounces

Coconut oil, .25 cup

Eggs, three

Pumpkin seeds, one third cup

Walnuts, chopped, one third cup

Baking powder, one tablespoon

Pumpkin pie spice, two tablespoons

Flaxseed, one half cup

Coconut flour, one and one quarter cups

Almond flour, one and one quarter cups

Psyllium husk powder, ground, two tablespoons

Salt, one teaspoon

Directions

Heat oven to 400. Use the lard to grease a nine by nine pan. Add the baking powder, pumpkin pie spice, nuts, psyllium husk powder, flaxseed, both flours, salt, and seeds into a bowl and mix together well. Use a separate bowl to cream together the oil, pumpkin puree, and egg. Gently pour this mixture into the dry ingredients and fold both together until all of the ingredients are well moistened. Spoon this entire mixture into the greased baking pan and bake it for one hour. Allow the bread to cool completely.

When the bread is done beat together the cream and eggs with the pepper and salt. Scramble the egg mix in the melted butter for five minutes, stirring constantly and then mix in the chili powder. Slice off two slices of the pumpkin bread and place them in the toaster to toast for three minutes. Butter the toasted pumpkin bread and lay each slice on a plate. Top each slice with the kale and the smoked salmon. Place the eggs on top of this and sprinkle with the chives.

Nutrition per serving:

Calories 678, 3 grams net carbs, 55 grams fat, 41 grams protein

Shrimp Deviled Eggs

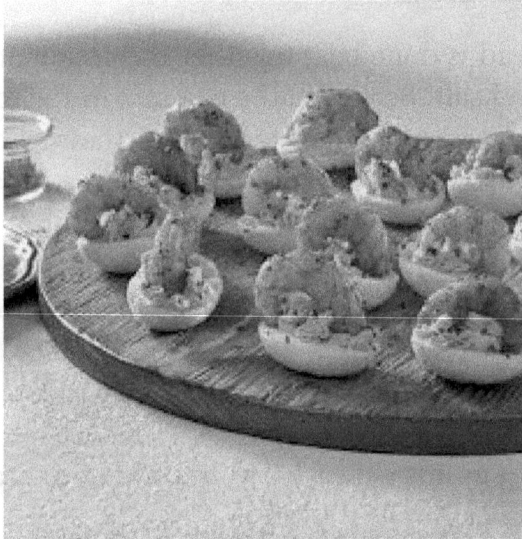

Preparation time: 5 minutes

Cooking time: 30 minutes

Serves four

Ingredients:

Chives, chopped, one teaspoon

Mayonnaise, one quarter cup

Eggs, four, hard boiled

Dill sprigs, eight fresh

Tabasco sauce, one teaspoon

Shrimp, peeled and deveined, eight large fully cooked*

Salt, one half teaspoon

White pepper, one half teaspoon

Directions

Carefully peel the chilled hard-boiled eggs and then cut them in half the long way and remove the yolks. Put the yolks into a bowl and use a dinner fork to gently mash the yolks and then add the Tabasco, salt, and mayonnaise. Mix all of this together well and then carefully spoon the mixture back into the egg whites. Top each egg with one cooked shrimp and a sprig of dill.

*Shrimp are sold whole or peeled and deveined. You can peel them yourself and remove the vein but the cost difference to buy them already peeled and deveined (P & D) in very small and worth the price.

Nutrition per serving:

Calories 163, .5 grams net carbs, 15 grams fat, 7 grams protein

Scrambled Eggs with Halloumi Cheese

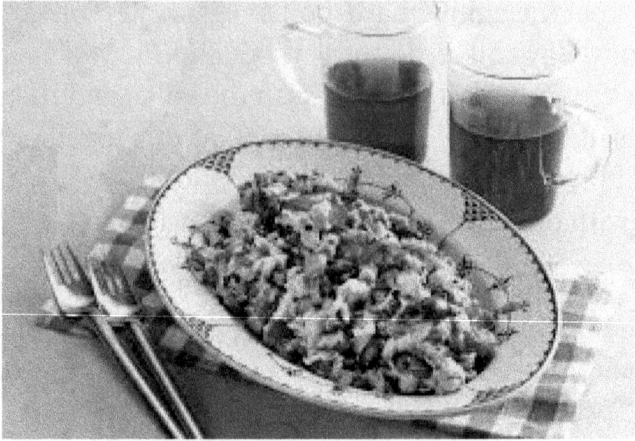

Preparation time: 5 minutes

Cooking time: 30 minutes

Serves two

Ingredients:

Eggs, four

Bacon, four slices

Salt, one half teaspoon

Black pepper, one teaspoon

Chili powder, one quarter teaspoon

Black olives, pitted if needed, one half cup

Parsley, fresh, one half cup chop fine

Scallions, two

Olive oil, two tablespoons

Halloumi cheese, diced from a block, three ounces

Directions

Chop finely the bacon and the cheese. Fry the bacon and the cheese with the scallions in the olive oil for five minutes. While this mixture is frying beat the eggs well with the parsley, pepper, chili powder, and salt. Dump the egg mix onto the bacon cheese mix in the skillet and scramble all together for three minutes while stirring constantly. Add in the olives and cook for three more minutes.

Nutrition per serving:

Calories 667, 4 grams carbs, 59 grams fat, 28 grams protein

Coconut Porridge

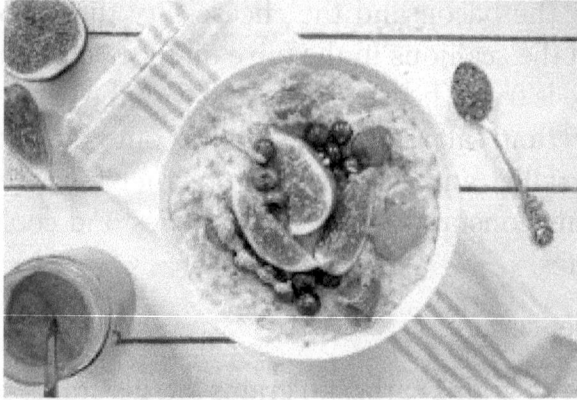

Preparation time: 5 minutes

Cooking time: 30 minutes

Serves one

Ingredients:

Egg, one

Salt, one quarter teaspoon

Coconut oil, one tablespoon

Coconut cream, four tablespoons

Psyllium husk powder, ground, one half teaspoon

Coconut flour, one tablespoon

Directions

Pour all of the ingredients listed into a pan and mix together well. Cook this mixture over very low heat while stirring constantly until the mixture is the thickness that you desire. Serve the porridge with a spoonful of coconut milk or heavy whipping cream and a few frozen or fresh berries if you like.

Nutrition per serving:

Calories 486, 4 grams net carbs, 49 grams fat, 9 grams protein

Western Omelet

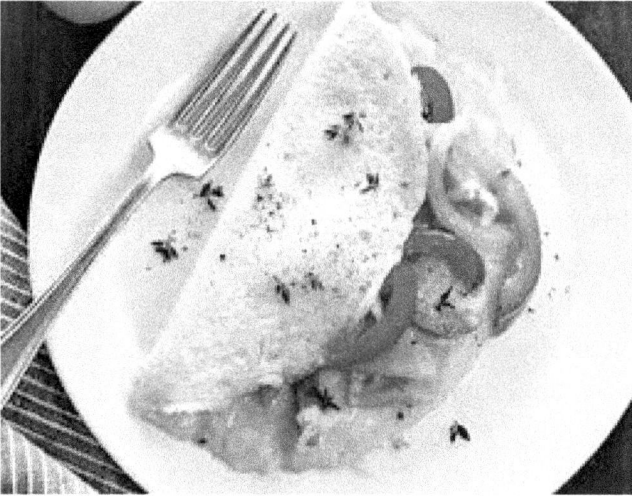

Preparation time: 5 minutes

Cooking time: 30 minutes

Serves two

Ingredients:

Eggs, six

Smoked deli ham, five ounces diced small

Butter, two tablespoons

Green bell pepper, one-half cup finely chopped

Yellow onion, one-quarter cup finely chopped

Shredded sharp cheddar cheese, three ounces

Sour cream, two tablespoons

Salt, one half teaspoon

Black pepper, one teaspoon

Chives, chopped, one tablespoon

Thyme, one quarter teaspoon

Directions

Cream together the eggs and the sour cream together until they are fluffy and season this mix with salt, chives, thyme, and pepper. Sprinkle in just half of the shredded cheese and mix it together well. Cook the peppers, onion, and ham in the melted butter for five minutes while stirring often. Dump the egg mixture carefully over the ham mixture in the skillet and cook for an additional five minutes just sitting still, do not stir. Sprinkle the remainder of the shredded cheese onto the omelet and carefully fold it in half and fry for five more minutes, two and one-half minutes per side.

Nutrition per serving:

Calories 702, 6 grams net carbs, 58 grams fat, 40 grams protein

Mushroom Omelet

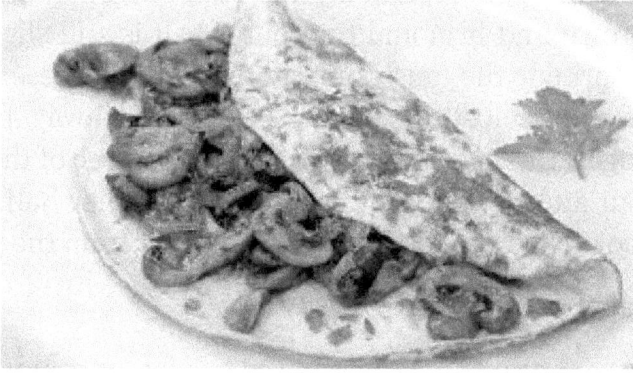

Preparation time: 5 minutes

Cooking time: 30 minutes

Serves one

Ingredients:

Eggs, three

Shredded cheese any style, one ounce

Mushrooms, one half cup

Yellow onion, diced fine, one quarter cup

Salt, one half teaspoon

White pepper, one quarter teaspoon

Rosemary, one half teaspoon

Butter, one tablespoon

Directions

Break the eggs into a bowl carefully and season them with the pepper, salt, and rosemary. Use a fork or a hand mixer to beat the eggs until they are well mixed and slightly frothy. Pour the egg mixture into the melted butter into the pan. Let the omelet cook over medium heat until the half-inch outer edge has begun to look brown and firm and the center half is still slightly raw and wet. Sprinkle the mushrooms, onions, and cheese onto the omelet, staying mostly near the center and away from the cooked edges. Use a spatula to work the edges free of the omelet off the pan and flip one side over onto the other half. Let the omelet cook five more minutes and remove it from the pan.

Nutrition per omelet:

Calories 510, 4 grams net carbs, 43 grams fat, 25 grams protein

Frittata with Fresh Spinach

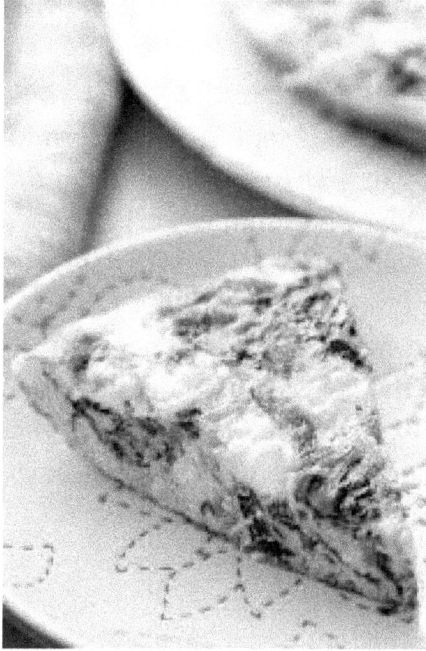

Preparation time: 5 minutes

Cooking time: 30 minutes

Serves four

Ingredients:

Eggs, eight

Heavy whipping cream, one cup

Salt, one teaspoon

Black pepper, one teaspoon

Rosemary, one half teaspoon

Thyme, one quarter teaspoon

Shredded sharp cheddar cheese, five ounces

Spinach, fresh, one cup washed and dried

Butter, two tablespoons

Directions

Heat oven to 350. Use one tablespoon of lard to grease a nine by nine-inch baking pan. Use one tablespoon of the butter to fry the bacon in a skillet over medium heat. When the bacon is crispy place the cleaned spinach in the skillet and cooks it until the spinach wilts. The bacon will break into pieces while you are stirring it with the spinach. During the time the bacon is cooking beat the eggs and the heavy cream together in a small bowl. Pour this mix into the baking pan, then add in the spinach and bacon mix and sprinkle all over the top with the sharp cheddar cheese. Bake for thirty minutes and serve hot.

Nutrition per serving:

Calories 661, 4 grams net carbs, 59 grams fat, 27 grams protein

Cauliflower Hash Browns

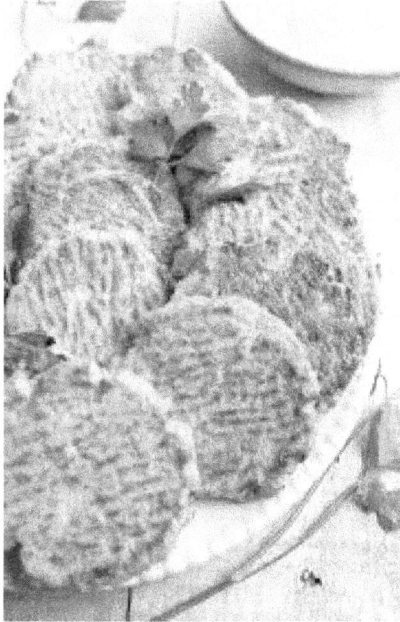

Preparation time: 5 minutes

Cooking time: 30 minutes

Serves four

Ingredients:

Eggs, three well beaten

Butter, four tablespoons

Yellow onion, one half grated

Black pepper, one teaspoon

Salt, one teaspoon

Cauliflower, one head

Directions

Wash and rinse the cauliflower and let drain well and then pat it dry. Grate the raw cauliflower finely using a hand grater or a food processor. Dump the finely grated cauliflower into a bowl and add the salt, pepper, egg, and onion. Mix all of this together very well. Form the grated cauliflower mixture into pancake shapes and fry them in the melted butter five minutes on each side. If they do not fry long enough, they will break apart when you flip them or remove them from the pan, so do not try to rush them.

Nutrition per serving:

Calories 282, 5 grams net carbs, 26 grams fat, 7 grams protein

Salmon Filled Avocado

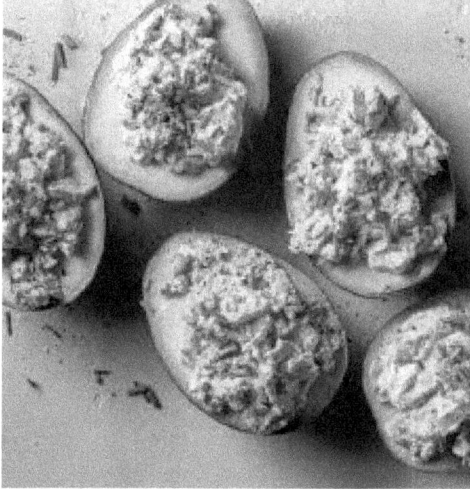

Preparation time: 5 minutes

Cooking time: 50 minutes

Serves two

Ingredients:

Avocados, two

Lemon juice, two tablespoons

Salt, one half teaspoon

Black pepper, one teaspoon

Sour cream, one cup

Smoked salmon, six ounces

Directions

Gently peel the raw avocados and cut them in half the long way and then remove the pit. Spoon the sour cream into the holes where the pit was and place the smoked salmon on top of the sour cream. Drizzle on the lemon juice and then season to taste with the salt and the pepper.

Nutrition per serving:

Calories 911, 6 grams net carbs, 71 grams fat, 58 grams protein

Rutabaga Fritters with Avocado

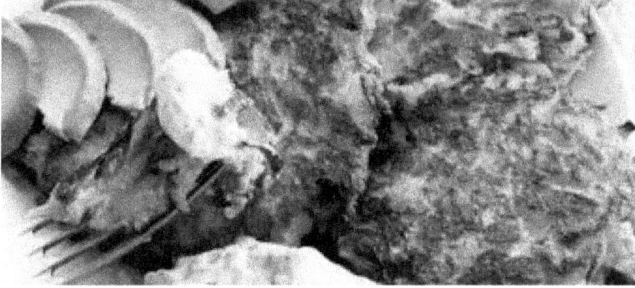

Preparation time: 5 minutes

Cooking time: 50 minutes

Serves four

Ingredients:

MAYONNAISE DRESSING

Ranch seasoning, one tablespoon

Mayonnaise, one cup

FRITTERS

Eggs, four

Butter, for frying, four tablespoons

Rutabaga, fifteen ounces

Pepper, one half teaspoon

Salt, one half teaspoon

Halloumi cheese, eight ounces

Turmeric, one quarter teaspoon

Coconut flour, three tablespoons

Serve with avocado slices and leafy greens of your choice

Directions

Heat oven to 250. Rinse the rutabaga well and peel it. Grate the rutabaga finely using a food processor or a hand grater. Use the same process for shredding the cheese. Use a large bowl to mix the coconut flour with the grated rutabaga, pepper, salt, cheese, turmeric, and eggs and let this mixture stand for ten minutes. Form the mixture into twelve equal-sized patties and fry them, three or four at a time, in the melted butter over medium heat. Fry the patties for five minutes on each side. Put the already cooked patties in the oven to keep them warm while you are cooking the rest. Top with the ranch dressing to serve.

Nutrition per serving:

Calories 1211, 14 grams net carbs, 113 grams fat, 25 grams protein

Bacon Mushroom Breakfast Casserole

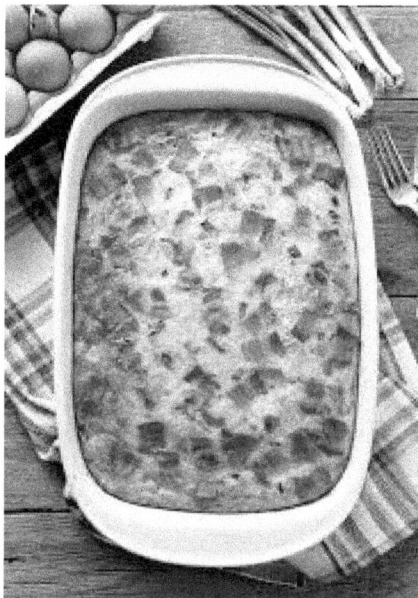

Preparation time: 5 minutes

Cooking time: 50 minutes

Serves four

Ingredients:

Eggs, eight

Bacon, twelve ounces

Heavy whipping cream, one cup

Butter, two tablespoons

Salt, one teaspoon

Pepper, one teaspoon

Cheddar cheese, shredded, five ounces

Mushrooms, six ounces

Directions

Heat oven to 400. Rinse and dry the mushrooms and chop them. Chop the bacon into bite-size pieces. Fry the bacon bits and the mushrooms in the butter for five minutes over medium heat. Use one tablespoon of lard to grease a nine by thirteen-inch baking dish and add the mushroom and bacon mixture to it. Beat the cream with the eggs, cheese, pepper, and salt in a bowl and pour into the baking dish on top of the bacon and mushrooms. Bake this for forty minutes.

Nutrition per serving:

Calories 876, 6 grams net carbs, 81 grams fat, 31 grams protein

Baked Eggs

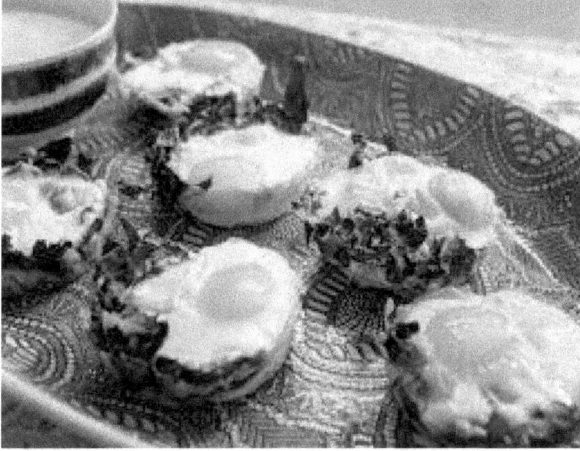

Preparation time : 5 minutes

Cooking time: 50 minutes

Serves one

Ingredients:

Eggs, two

Ground pork, three ounces cooked

Shredded cheddar cheese, two ounces

Directions

Heat oven to 400. Use one tablespoon of lard to grease a small baking pan about a five by five-inch. Lay the cooked ground pork in the pan. Then crack both eggs and over the top of the cooked pork. Sprinkle all over the top with shredded cheese and bake for fifteen minutes.

Nutrition per serving:

Calories 509, 2 grams net carbs, 36 grams fat, 42 grams protein

Keto Blueberry Muffins

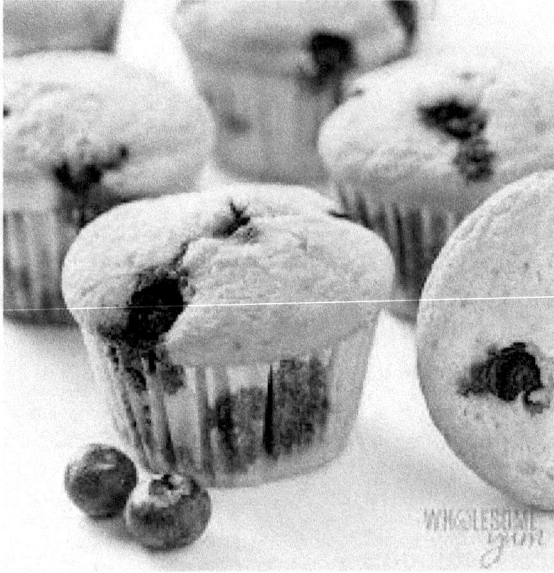

Preparation time: 5 minutes

Cooking time: 50 minute s

Serves six to twelve

Ingredients:

Lemon zest, one tablespoon

Blueberries, fresh, one half cup

Vanilla, one teaspoon

Eggs, three large

Almond milk, unsweetened

Butter, one-third cup melted

Salt, one half teaspoon

Baking soda, one half teaspoon

Baking powder, one and one half teaspoon

Almond flour, two and one half cups

Directions

Heat oven to 350. Use paper or foil liners to line all twelve cups of a twelve cup muffin pan. Use a large bowl to mix the almond flour with the salt, baking soda, and baking powder. Then mix in the vanilla, eggs, almond milk, and melted butter just until the dry ingredients are wet. Then gently fold in the lemon zest and the blueberries until they are mixed evenly into the batter. Divide the batter among the twelve cups until all of the batter is used. Bake the muffins twenty to twenty-five minutes until a knife inserted in the center of one comes out clean. Let them cool slightly before eating.

Nutrition per muffin:

Calories 229, 4 grams net carbs, 19 grams fat, 8 grams protein

Taco Breakfast Skillet

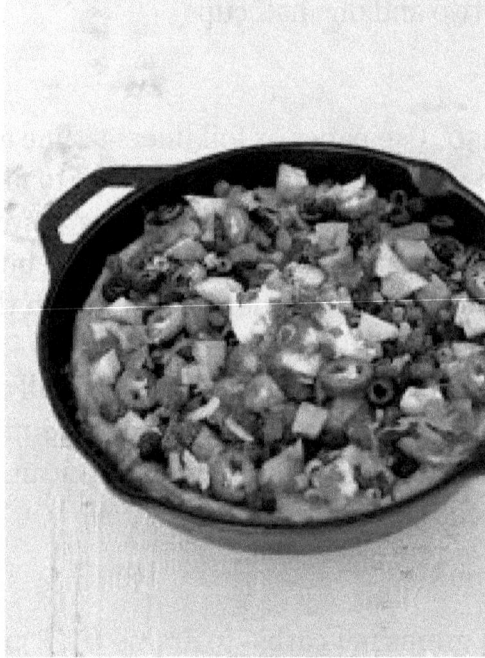

Preparation time: 5 minutes

Cooking time: 50 minutes

Serves six

Ingredients:

Cilantro, two tablespoons fresh torn

Jalapeno, one sliced

Salsa, one quarter cup

Green onions, two sliced thin

Black olives, one quarter cup sliced

Avocado, one medium peeled, pitted, cubed

Roma tomato, one diced

Heavy cream, one quarter cup

Sharp cheddar cheese, shredded, one and one-half cup divided

Eggs, ten

Water, two-thirds cup

Taco seasoning, four tablespoons

Ground beef, one pound

Directions

Heat oven to 375. Cook the ground beef until fully cooked in a large skillet over medium heat. Drain off the excess fat. Add the taco seasoning and the water to the meat back in the skillet. Turn the heat down to low and let the mix simmer until the water has almost disappeared and the seasoning is coating the meat, for about five minutes. Beat the eggs together well in a large bowl and add the heavy cream and one cup of the cheese and mix well. Pour the meat mixture into a greased nine by nine baking dish and pour the egg mixture on top. Bake this for thirty minutes. Cover the mix with the rest of the shredded cheese, green onion, olives, tomato, and avocado. Serve with the cilantro, jalapeno, salsa, and sour cream on the side for garnish.

Nutrition per serving:

Calories 563, 9 grams carbs, 44 grams fat, 32 grams protein

Cream Cheese Pancakes

Preparation time: 5 minutes

Cooking time: 50 minutes

Serves one

Ingredients:

Cinnamon, one teaspoon

Eggs, two

Cream cheese, two ounces

Butter, two tablespoons

Directions

Make a smooth batter by mixing well all of the ingredients. Let the batter rest for five minutes. Pour in one-quarter of the batter into melted butter in a skillet over medium heat. Cook all of the pancakes for about two to three minutes on each side. Serve them with fruit if desired.

Nutrition info:

Calories 344, 3 grams net carbs, 29 grams fat, 17 grams protein

Keto Cloud Bread

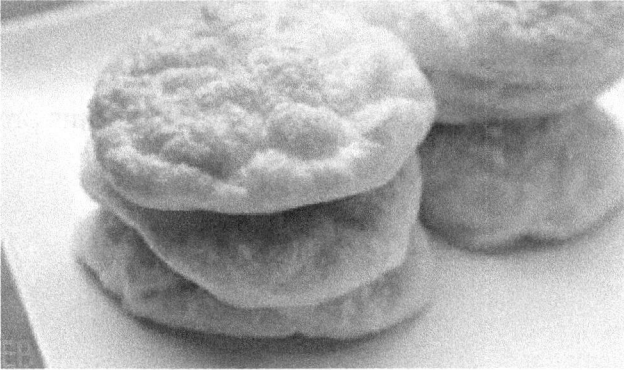

This recipe is perfect for any meal. Have it for breakfast with a bit of keto strawberry jam as an occasional treat. And look for the strawberry jam recipe in this book.

Preparation time: 5 minutes

Cooking time: 50 minutes

Ingredients:

Salt, one quarter teaspoon

Cream of tartar, one quarter teaspoon

Cream cheese, three tablespoons at room temperature

Eggs, three at room temperature

Directions

Heat oven to 350. Cover two cookie sheets with parchment paper. Separate the three eggs and put the whites in one bowl and the yolks in another. Blend the cream cheese into the egg yolks. Mix until there are no yellow streaks remaining. Spoon the mixture onto the parchment paper covered cookie sheets in mounds about three inches across and one half inch high. Bake for thirty minutes on the middle oven rack. Allow the bread to cool completely before using.

Nutrition per piece:

Calories 35, .4 grams carbs, 2.8-gram fat, 2.2 grams protein

Chapter 8:
Lunch

Vegan Tuna Salad

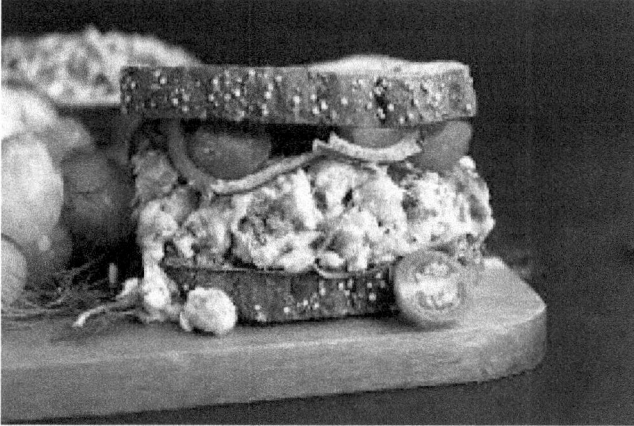

Preparation time: 5 minutes

Cooking time: 55 minutes

Servings: 6

Ingredients:

2 cans chickpeas

1 tablespoon prepared yellow mustard

2 tablespoons vegan mayonnaise

1 tablespoon jarred capers

2 tablespoons pickle relish

½ cup chopped celery

Directions

1. In a medium bowl, combine chickpeas, mustard, vegan mayo, and mustard. Pulse in a food processor or mash with a potato masher until the mixture is partially smooth with some chunks.

2. Add the remaining ingredients to the chickpea mixture and mix until combined.

3. Serve immediately or refrigerate until ready to serve.

Nutritional info: Calories: 170, Fat: 18g, Protein: 15g, Carbs: 1.8g

Veggie Wrap with Apples and Spicy Hummus

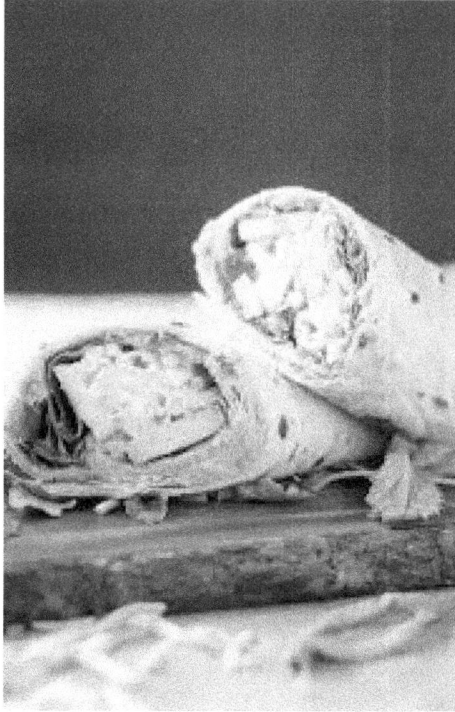

Preparation time: 5 minutes

Cooking time: 40 minutes

Servings: 6

Ingredients:

1 tortilla of your choice: flour, corn, gluten-free, etc.

3-4 tablespoons of your favorite spicy hummus (a plain hummus mixed with salsa is good, too!)

A few leaves of your favorite leafy greens

¼ apple sliced thin

½ cup broccoli slaw (store-bought or homemade are both good)

½ teaspoon lemon juice

2 teaspoons dairy-free, plain, unsweetened yogurt

Salt and pepper to taste

Directions

1. Mix broccoli slaw with lemon juice and yogurt. Add pepper and salt to taste and mix well.

2. Lay tortilla flat.

3. Spread hummus all over the tortilla.

4. Lay down leafy greens on hummus.

5. On one half, pile broccoli slaw over lettuce. Place apples on top of the slaw.

6. Starting with the half with slaw and apples, roll tortilla tightly.

7. Cut in half if desired and enjoy!

Nutritional info: Calories: 110, Fat: 8g, Protein: 15g, Carbs: 8g

Turmeric Rack of Lamb

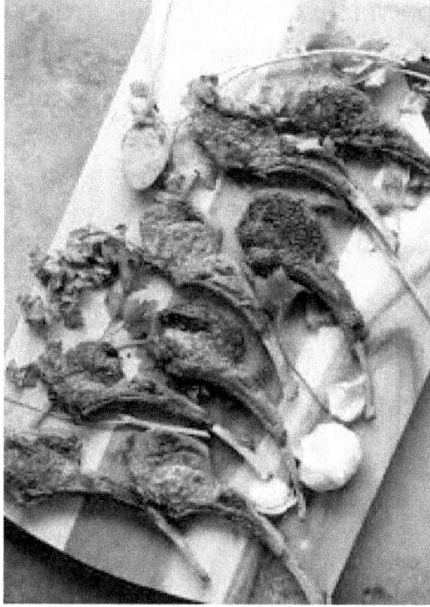

Preparation time: 15 minutes

Cooking time: 16 minute s

Servings:4

Ingredients:

13 oz rack of lamb

1 tablespoon ground turmeric

½ teaspoon chili flakes

3 tablespoons olive oil

1 tablespoon balsamic vinegar

1 teaspoon salt

½ teaspoon peppercorns

¾ cup of water

Directions

In the shallow bowl, mix up together ground turmeric, chili flakes, olive oil, balsamic vinegar, salt, and peppercorns.

Brush the rack of lamb with the oily mixture generously.

After this, preheat grill to 380F.

Place the rack of lamb in the grill and cook it for 8 minutes from each side.

The cooked rack of lamb should have a light crunchy crust.

Nutritional info: Calories: 190, Fat: 28g, Protein: 15g, Carbs: 8g

Sausage Casserole

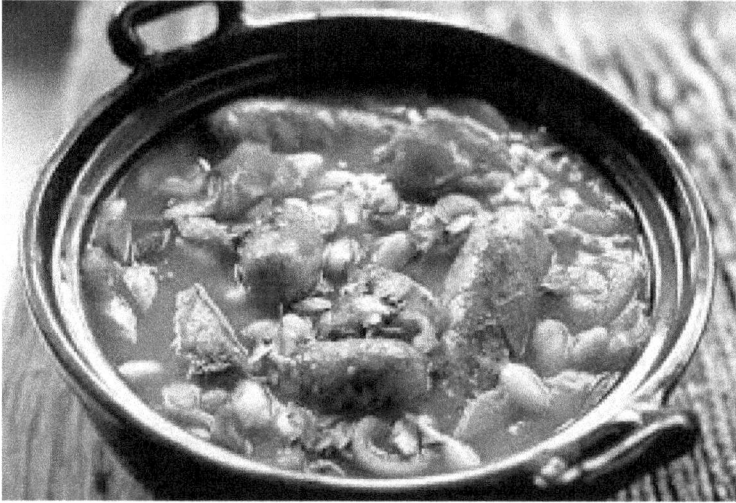

Preparation time: 10 minutes

Cooking time: 35 minutes

Servings:6

Ingredients:

2 jalapeno peppers, sliced

5 oz Cheddar cheese, shredded

9 oz sausages, chopped

1 tablespoon olive oil

½ cup spinach, chopped

½ cup heavy cream

½ teaspoon salt

Directions

Brush the casserole mold with the olive oil from inside.

Then put the chopped sausages in the casserole mold in one layer.

Add chopped spinach and sprinkle it with salt.

After this, add sliced jalapeno pepper.

Then make the layer of shredded Cheddar cheese.

Pour the heavy cream over the cheese.

Preheat the oven to 355F.

Transfer the casserole in the oven and cook it for 35 minutes.

Use the kitchen torch to make the crunchy cheese crust of the casserole.

Nutritional info: Calories: 150, Fat: 18g, Protein: 15g, Carbs: 1.8g

Cajun Pork Sliders

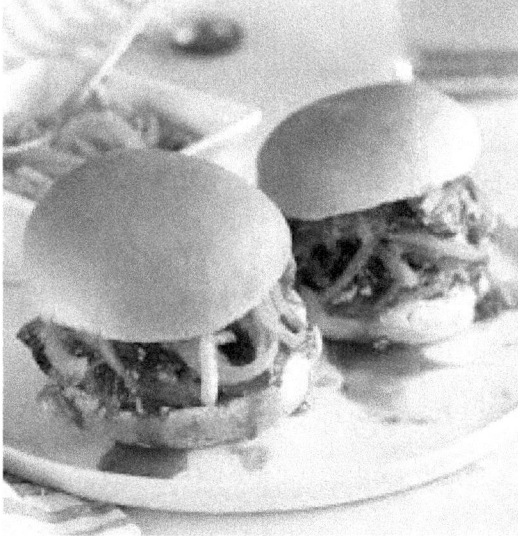

Preparation time: 10 minutes

Cooking time: 45 minutes

Servings:4

Ingredients:

4 low carb bread slices

14 oz pork loin

2 tablespoons Cajun spices

1 tablespoon olive oil

1/3 cup water

1 teaspoon tomato sauce

Directions

Rub the pork loin with Cajun spices and place in the skillet.

Add olive oil and roast it over the high heat for 5 minutes from each side.

After this, transfer the meat in the saucepan, add tomato sauce and water.

Stir gently and close the lid.

Simmer the meat for 35 minutes.

Slice the cooked pork loin.

Place the pork sliders over the bread slices and transfer in the serving plates.

Nutritional info: Calories: 70, Fat: 18g, Protein: 15g, Carbs: 1.8g

Mac and Cheese Bites

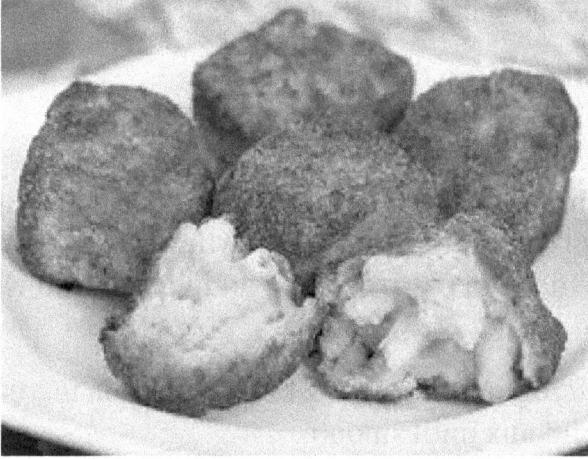

Preparation time: 5 minutes

Cooking time: 50 minutes

Servings: 5

Ingredients:

1 ½ cups uncooked macaroni (gluten-free will work if needed)

1 medium onion, chopped (can substitute with 1 medium yellow pepper if you don't care for onions.)

1 clove garlic, chopped

2 tablespoons cornstarch, or arrowroot powder

1 cup non-dairy milk

½ teaspoon smoked paprika (can substitute for chipotle powder)

1 teaspoon lemon juice or apple cider vinegar

½ cup nutritional yeast

1 teaspoon salt

Directions

1. Preheat your oven to 350 degrees Fahrenheit.

2. Prepare the muffin tin with liners.

3. Prepare macaroni according to Directions.

4. While macaroni is cooking, sauté garlic and onion (or substitute of choice) until it is just starting to turn golden brown. This can be done in a dry pan, but adding some oil will work as well.

5. Add garlic, onion, and all other non-macaroni ingredients into a blender and mix until smooth.

6. Drain the macaroni and return to the pan.

7. Pour sauce over macaroni and stir well.

8. Spoon mixture into muffin tin, stirring occasionally in between such an equal amount of sauce goes in each cup.

9. Push down tops with the back of a spoon.

10. Bake in the oven for 30 min.

11. Serve once cooled.

Nutritional info: Calories: 100, Fat: 10g, Protein: 12g, Carbs: 1.8g

Chick'n Salad with Cranberries and Pistachios

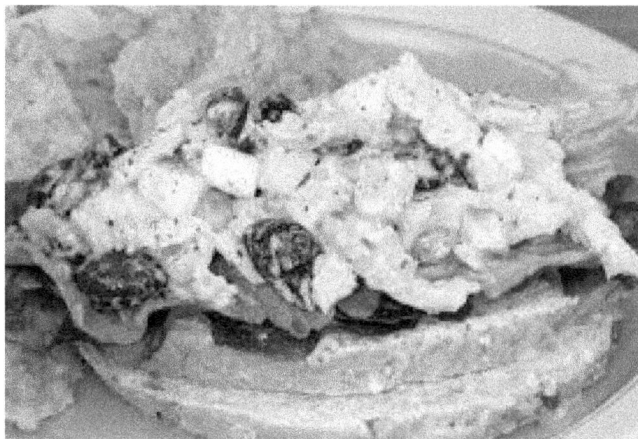

Preparation time: 5 minutes

Cooking time: 80 minutes

Servings: 6

Ingredients:

1 ½ cups dry soy curls (textured vegetable protein)

2 dashes apple cider vinegar

½ cup diced granny smith apples (approx. 1 small apple)

¼ cup shelled pistachios, chopped

½ cup dried cranberries

5-6 tablespoons veganaise (adjust depending on how creamy you would like the salad to be)

1 teaspoon of sea salt

A pinch of thyme

Directions

1. Soak soy curls in warm water for 10 min. Squeeze excess water out of them and roughly chop larger pieces. Set aside.

2. While soy curls are soaking, mix diced apple and vinegar. Drain any excess liquid.

3. Combine apples with all other ingredients in large bowl until ingredients are evenly mixed. Add seasoning to taste. Chill for at least 30 minutes. Serve as desired.

Nutritional info: Calories: 200, Fat: 20g, Protein: 15g, Carbs: 15g

Tuna Casserole

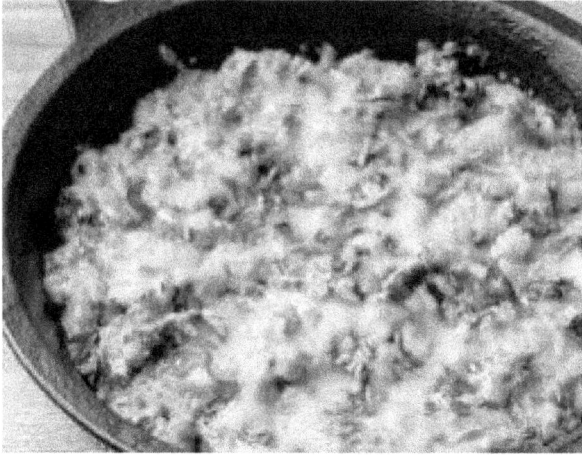

Preparation time: 5 minutes

Cooking time: 50 minutes

Serves four

Ingredients:

Tuna in oil, sixteen ounces, drained

Butter, two tablespoons

Salt, one half teaspoon

Black pepper, one teaspoon

Chili powder, one teaspoon

Celery, six stalks

Green bell pepper, one

Yellow onion, one

Parmesan cheese, grated, four ounces

Mayonnaise, one cup

Directions

Heat the oven to 400. Chop the onion, bell pepper, and celery very fine and fry in the melted butter for five minutes. Stir together with the chili powder, parmesan cheese, tuna, and mayonnaise. Use lard to grease an eight by eight-inch or nine by a nine-inch baking pan. Add the tuna mixture into the fried vegetables and spoon the mix into the baking pan. Bake it for twenty minutes.

Nutrition per serving:

Calories 953, 5 grams net carbs, 83 grams fat, 43 grams protein

White Fish with Curry and Coconut

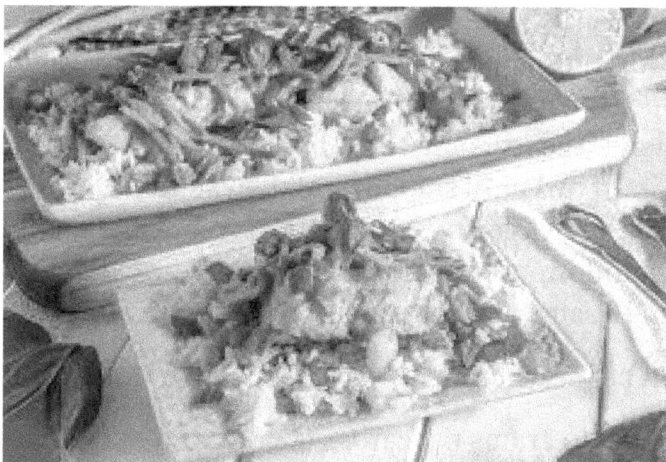

Preparation time: 5 minutes

Cooking time: 40 minutes

Serves four

Ingredients:

Whitefish or salmon, twenty-five ounces approximately in four pieces

Salt, one teaspoon

Pepper, one teaspoon

Broccoli or cauliflower, two cups

Cilantro, fresh, chopped, one half cup

Coconut cream, fourteen ounces

Curry paste, green or red, two tablespoons

Butter or ghee, four tablespoons

Lard to grease baking pan

Directions

Heat the oven to 400. Use two tablespoons of lard to grease a nine by thirteen-inch baking pan and lay the fish pieces in it. Salt and pepper the fish pieces and lay a pat of butter on top of each slice. Blend the coconut cream, curry paste, and chopped cilantro in a bowl until smooth and then spoon this mix over the fish. Bake the fish for twenty minutes. While the fish is baking cut the cauliflower or the broccoli into bite-size florets and then boil them in salt water for five minutes.

Nutrition per serving:

Calories 880, 9 grams net carbs, 75 grams fat, 42 grams protein

Creamy Fish Casserole

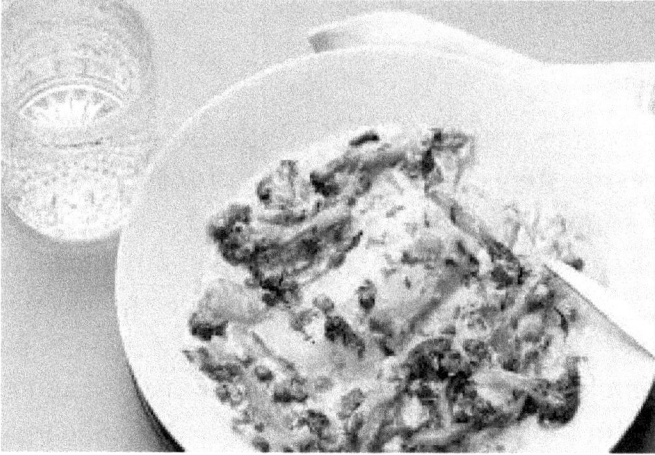

Preparation time: 5 minutes

Cooking time: 40 minutes

Serves four

Ingredients:

Whitefish, twenty-five ounces approximately, cut into four serving pieces

Capers, small, two tablespoons

Scallions, six

Broccoli, sixteen ounces

Butter, three tablespoons

Dijon mustard, one tablespoon

Heavy whipping cream, one and one quarter cups

Parsley, dried, one tablespoon

Black pepper, one teaspoon

Salt, one teaspoon

Olive oil, two tablespoons

Directions

Heat the oven to 400. Rinse and dry the broccoli and cut it into florets leaving stems on. Use the oil to fry the broccoli for five minutes stirring occasionally. Add in the scallions and the capers. Fry for three minutes, stirring once. Use butter to grease a nine by thirteen-inch baking dish. Place the veggies in the baking dish. Lay the fish in on top of the veggies. In a small bowl mix the parsley, whipping cream, and the mustard and pour this mix on top of the vegetables and fish in the baking pan. Bake for thirty minutes. Lay six pats of butter on top in random places and let it melt before serving. Serve with a bowl of leafy greens.

Nutrition per serving:

Calories 822, 8 grams net carbs, 69 grams fat, 41 grams protein

Spinach and Goat Cheese Pie

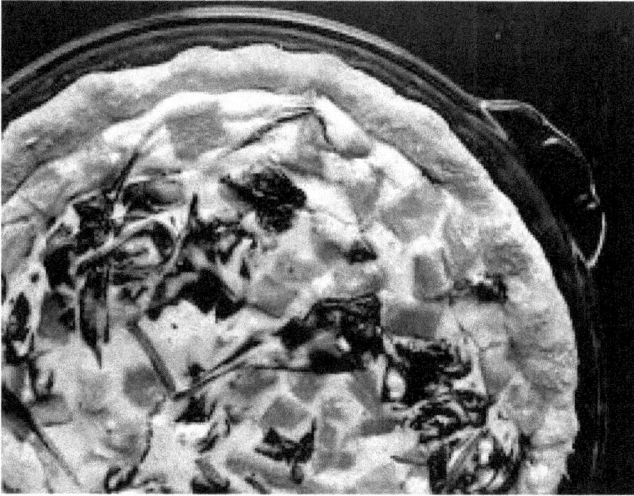

Preparation time: 5 minutes

Cooking time: 40 minutes

Serves six

Ingredients:

EGG BATTER

Sour cream, one cup

Eggs, five

Salt, one half teaspoon

Black pepper, one teaspoon

PIE CRUST

Almond flour, one and one half cups

Butter, two tablespoons

Salt, one half teaspoon

Egg, one

Psyllium husk powder, ground, one tablespoon

Sesame seeds

GOAT CHEESE AND SPINACH FILLING

Spinach, fresh, eight ounces

Goat cheese, six ounces sliced

Salt, one half teaspoon

Black pepper, one teaspoon

Cheddar cheese, shredded, one half cup

Nutmeg, ground, one half teaspoon

Garlic, one clove

Butter, two tablespoons

Directions

Heat the oven to 350. Use a fork to mix the ingredients for the dough until you make a ball of dough. Press this dough into a greased springform pan covering the bottom and the sides. Use a fork to poke holes randomly in the crust, about ten to fifteen sets. Bake the empty pie shell for ten minutes. Cream together the eggs, sour cream, salt, and pepper. Chop the garlic and the spinach fine. Fry the garlic and the spinach in the hot butter for five minutes stirring occasionally. Put this mix into the pie shell and sprinkle the grated cheese over the top. Pour the creamed egg mixture over all ingredients and place the goat cheese on top. Bake for forty-five minutes.

Nutrition per serving:

Calories 643, 4 grams net carbs, 58 grams fat, 24 grams protein

Avocado Pie

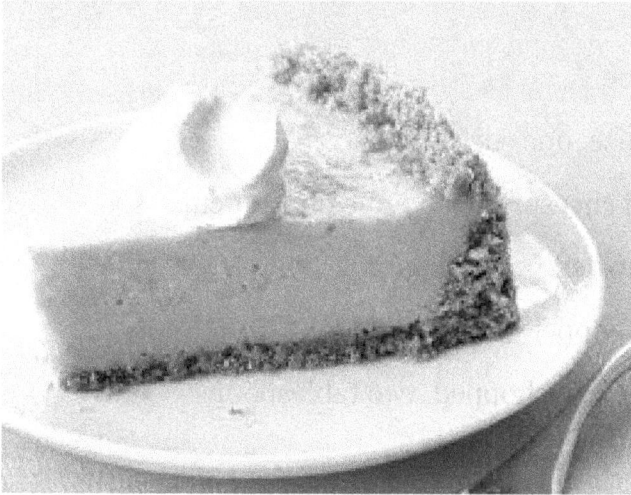

Preparation time: 5 minutes

Cooking time: 50 minutes

Serves four

Ingredients:

PIE CRUST

Coconut flour, four tablespoons

Almond flour, three-fourths of a cup

Psyllium husk powder, ground, one tablespoon

Sesame seeds, four tablespoons

Water, four tablespoons

Egg, one

Olive oil, three tablespoons

Salt, one quarter teaspoon

Baking powder, one teaspoon

FILLING

Eggs, three

Mayonnaise, one cup

Shredded cheese, one and one quarter cups

Onion powder, one teaspoon

Red chili pepper, one chop fine

Cilantro, fresh chopped, two tablespoons

Cream cheese, one half cup

Salt, one half teaspoon

Avocados, two ripe

Directions

Heat the oven to 350. Use a fork to mix the crust ingredients in a bowl or use a food processor to mix them. Use two tablespoons of lard to grease a deep pie pan. Lay the dough ball into the pie dish, using your fingers or a spatula to spread it all over the bottom of the pan and up the sides. Poke ten to fifteen sets of holes in the bottom with a dinner fork and bake the crust empty for ten minutes. Wash and peel the avocado and remove the pit, then dice the avocado. Clean the seeds out of the chili and dice it. Mix together the diced chili and the diced avocado with the rest of the ingredients. Spoon this mix into the pre-baked crust and bake all for an additional forty minutes.

Nutrition per serving:

Calories 1146, 9 grams net carbs, 109 grams fat, 26 grams protein

Tex Mex Stuffed Zucchini Boats

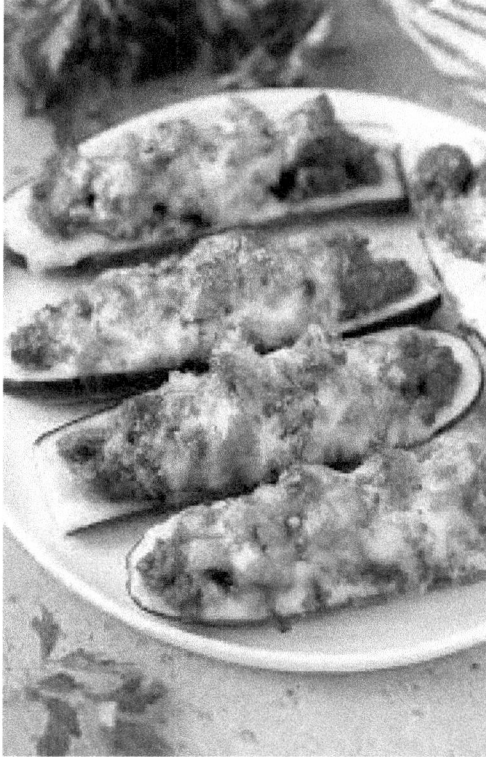

Preparation time: 5 minutes

Cooking time: 40 minutes

Serves four

Ingredients:

Ground beef, one pound

Zucchini, two medium-sized

Cilantro, fresh, chopped fine, one half cup

Cheddar cheese, shredded, one and one half cups

Olive oil, one tablespoon

Salt, one teaspoon

Tex Mex seasoning, two tablespoons

Olive oil or butter, two tablespoons

Directions

Heat the oven to 400. Cut both zucchinis in half down the length and remove the seeds but do not peel. Cook the ground beef in the olive oil until it is brown, about ten minutes. Stir in the salt and the Tex Mex seasoning and let this cook until all of the liquid has cooked away. Use two tablespoons of lard to grease a nine by thirteen-inch baking pan and lay the zucchini halves in it cut side up. Stir one-third of the shredded cheese into the meat mixture and add the cilantro. Fill the halves of the zucchini evenly with the meat and cheese mix. Use the rest of the shredded cheese to sprinkle on the top. Bake the zucchini boats for twenty minutes.

Nutrition per serving:

Calories 601, 6 grams net carbs, 49 grams fat, 33 grams protein

Brussel Sprouts and Hamburger Gratin

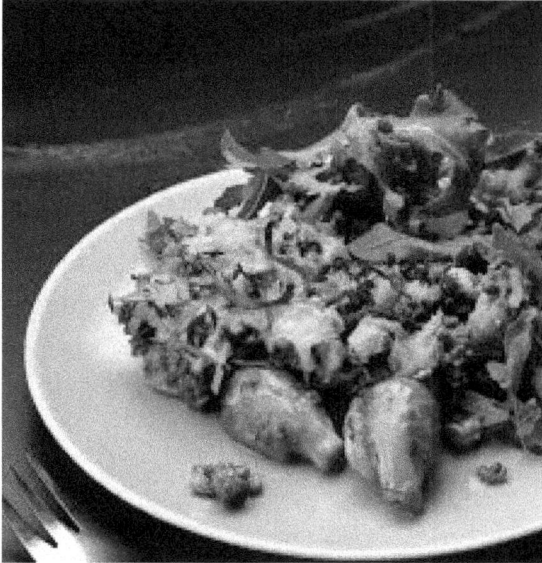

Preparation time: 5 minutes

Cooking time: 40 minutes

Serves four

Ingredients:

Ground beef, one pound

Bacon, eight ounces, diced small

Brussel sprouts, fifteen ounces, cut in half

Salt, one teaspoon

Black pepper, one teaspoon

Thyme, one half teaspoon

Cheddar cheese, shredded, one cup

Italian seasoning, one tablespoon

Sour cream, four tablespoons

Butter, two tablespoons

Directions

Heat the oven to 425. Fry bacon and Brussel sprouts in butter for five minutes. Stir in the sour cream and pour this mix into a greased eight by eight-inch baking pan. Cook the ground beef and season with the salt and pepper, then add this mix to the baking pan. Top with the herbs and the shredded cheese. Bake for twenty minutes.

Nutrition per serving:

Calories 770, 8 grams net carbs, 62 grams fat, 42 grams protein

SoyLime Roasted Tofu

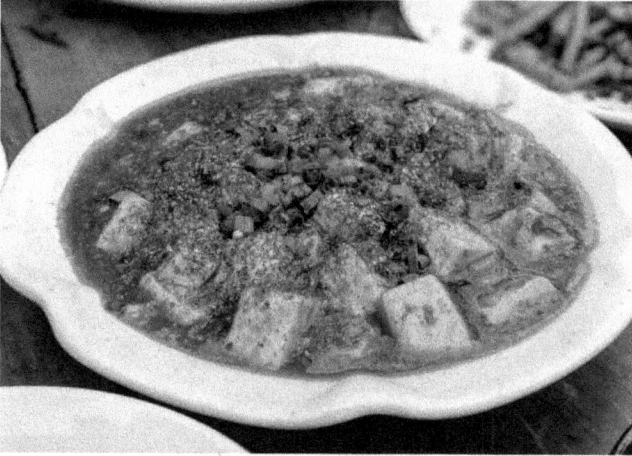

Preparation time: 15 minutes; Cook time: 1hour 35 minutes; Servings: 4

Ingredients

Extra-firm tofu, drained and cubed – 28 oz.

Reduced-sodium soy sauce – 2/3 cup

Lime juice – 2/3 cup

Sesame oil, toasted – 6 tablespoons.

Directions:

In a bowl, mix oil, lime juice, and sauce. Toss in tofu. Refrigerate for 1 hour to marinate.

Set oven to 450 degrees F

Remove tofu from marinade and spread on 2 baking sheets with some spacing between the pieces. Roast for 20 minutes as you turn halfway until golden brown.

Nutrition info: Calories: 163, Fat: 11g, Carbs: 2g, Protein: 19g

Chicken Nuggets

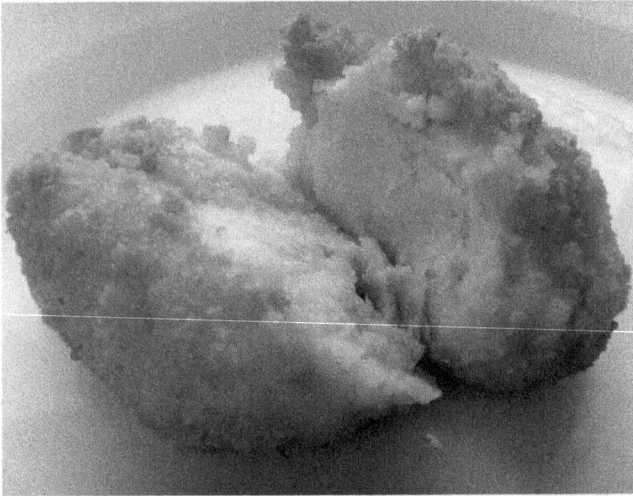

Preparation time: 5 minutes; Cook time: 20 minutes; Servings: 6

Ingredients:

Chicken, cooked - 2 cups

Cream Cheese - 8 oz.

Egg - 1

Almond Flour - ¼ cup

Garlic Salt - 1 teaspoon.

Directions:

While the chicken is still warm, set it in an electric mixer and shred. In case you are using leftover chicken, warm it up for a short period of time.

Once the shredding is done, add all the remaining ingredients and mix it up.

Drop scoops of the mixture onto a greased baking sheet, flatten it into a nugget shape.

Bake it for 13 minutes at 350 degrees, till they turn golden and cooked.

Enjoy when hot!

Nutritional info: Calories: 150, Fat: 18g, Protein: 15g, Carbs: 1.8g

Crab-Stuffed Avocado

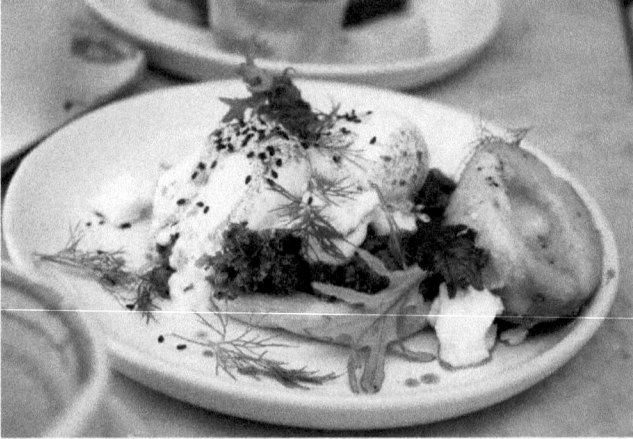

Preparation time: 10 minutes; Cook time: 5 minutes; Servings: 5

Ingredients:

Crab – 1 pound.

Avocado, ripe, pitted, peeled - 1

Onion, finely chopped - 2 tablespoons.

Cilantro, chopped - 2 tablespoons.

Salt

Pepper

Directions:

Place the crab in the Instant Pot and add a cup of water.

Set the lid in place and the vent should point to "Sealing."

Set the IP to manual and cook for 5 minutes.

Do quick pressure release.

Take the crab out and let it cool.

Extract the meat from the crab and discard the shells.

In a bowl, combine the crabmeat and stir in the rest of the ingredients.

Refrigerate.

Serve chilled.

Nutrition info: Calories: 149, Carbs: 4.7g, Protein: 13.2g, Fat: 15.3g

Thai Fish Curry

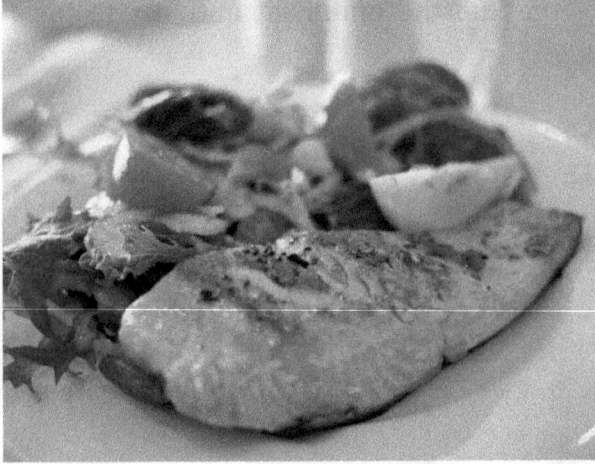

Preparation time: 5 minutes; Cook time: 10 minutes; Servings: 6

Ingredients

Olive oil - 1/3 cup

Salmon fillets - 1½ pounds.

Coconut milk, freshly squeezed - 2 cups

Curry powder - 2 tablespoons.

Cilantro chopped - ¼ cup

Directions:

In your instant pot, add in all ingredients. Apply a seasoning of pepper and salt.

Give a good stir.

Set the lid in place and the vent to point to "Sealing."

Set the IP to "Manual" and cook for 10 minutes.

Do quick pressure release.

Nutrition info: Calories: 470, Carbs: 5.6g, Protein: 25.5g, Fat: 39.8g

Avocado Grapefruit Salad

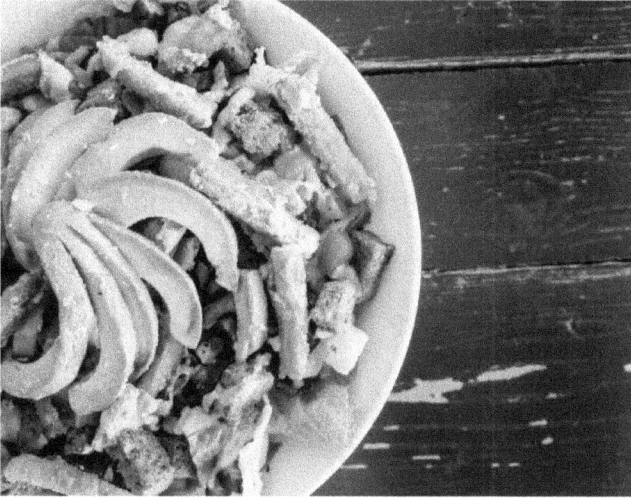

Preparation time: 5 minutes; Cook time: 20 minutes; Servings: 4

Ingredients:

Avocados, peeled, pitted and meat scooped - 2

Grapefruit, red, peeled - 1

Pomegranate seeds - ¼ cup

Shallots, minced - 1 tablespoon.

Olive oil - ¼ cup

Pomegranate juice - 1 tablespoon.

Salt

Pepper

Directions:

Squeeze some of the grapefruit to obtain the juice. Sprinkle over the avocados in a bowl. Spread over the remaining grapefruit and the pomegranate seeds.

In another bowl, mix olive oil, salt, pepper, pomegranate juice, and shallots. Sprinkle over the salad and enjoy.

Nutritional info: Calories: 335, Fat: 18g, Protein: 3g, Carbs: 28g

Garlic Herb Grilled Chicken Breast

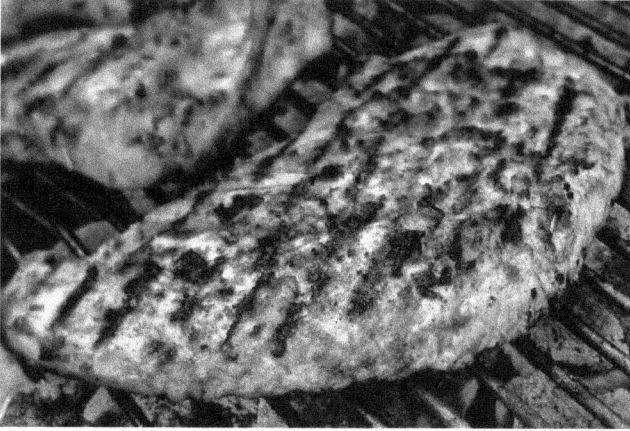

Preparation time: 7 minutes; Cook time: 20 minutes; Servings: 4

Ingredients:

Chicken Breasts, skinless and boneless - 1¼ pounds.

Olive oil - 2 teaspoons.

Garlic & Herb Seasoning Blend - 1 tablespoon.

Salt

Pepper

Directions:

Pat dry the chicken breasts, coat it with olive oil and season it with salt and pepper on both sides.

Season the chicken with garlic and herb seasoning or any other seasoning of your choice.

Turn the grill on and oil the grate.

Place the chicken on the hot grate and let it grill till the sides turn white.

Flip them over and let it cook again.

When the internal temperature is about 160 degree, it is most likely cooked.

Set aside for 15 minutes. Chop into pieces.

Nutritional info: Calories: 187, Fats: 6g, Protein: 32g, Carbs: 5g

Cajun Shrimp

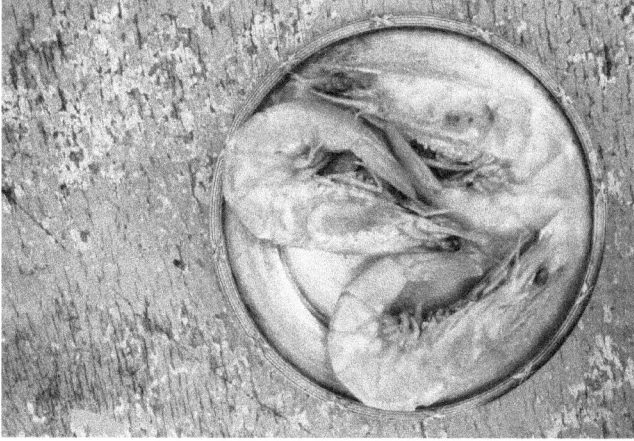

Preparation time: 10 minutes; Cook time: 5 minutes; Servings: 2

Ingredients

Tiger shrimp - 16

Corn starch - 2 tablespoons.

Cayenne pepper - 1 teaspoon.

Old bay seasoning – 1 teaspoon.

Salt

Pepper

Olive oil – 1 teaspoon.

Directions

Rinse the shrimp. Pat dry.

In a bowl, combine corn starch, cayenne pepper, old bay seasoning, salt, pepper. Stir.

In a bowl, add the shrimp. Drizzle olive oil over shrimp to lightly coat.

Dip the shrimp in seasoning, shake off any excess.

Preheat fryer to 375°F. Lightly spray cook basket with non-stick Keto cooking spray.

Transfer to fryer. Cook 5 minutes; shake after 2 minutes, until cooked thoroughly.

Serve on a platter.

Nutritional info: Calories: 127, Fat: 10g, Carbs: 3g, Protein: 7g

Sesame-Crusted Mahi-Mahi

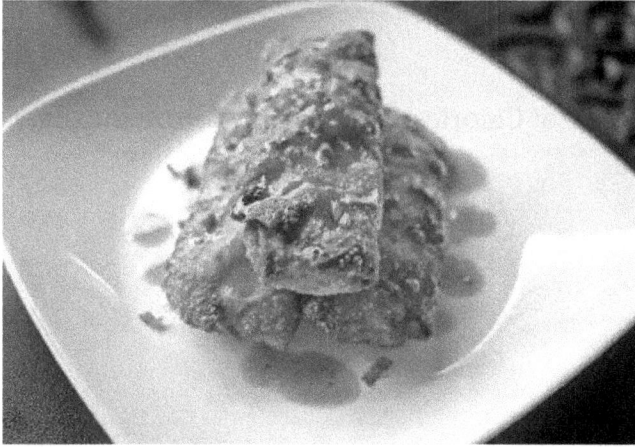

Preparation time: 5 minutes; Cook time: 13 minutes; Servings: 4

Ingredients:

Dijon mustard - 2 tablespoons.

Sour cream, low-fat – 1 tablespoon.

Sesame seeds - ½ cup

Olive oil - 2 tablespoons.

Lemon, wedged - 1

Mahi-mahi or sole filets - 4 (4 oz. each)

Directions:

Rinse filets and pat dry. In a bowl, mix sour cream and mustard. Spread this mixture on all sides of fish. Roll in sesame seeds to coat.

Heat olive oil in a large skillet over medium heat. Pan-fry fish, turning once, for 5–8 minutes or until fish flakes when tested with fork and sesame seeds are toasted. Serve immediately with lemon wedges.

Nutritional info: Calories: 282, Fat: 17g, Protein: 18g, Carbs: 5g

Country Chicken

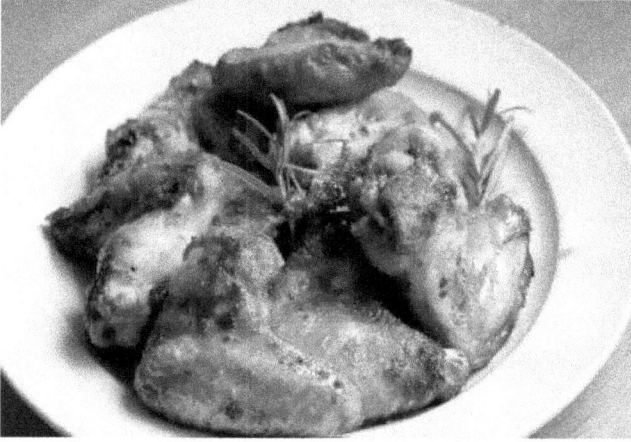

Preparation time: 10 minutes; Cook time: 15 minutes; Servings: 2

Ingredients

Chicken tenders, fresh, boneless skinless – ¾ pound.

Almond meal - ½ cup

Almond flour - ½ cup

Rosemary, dried - 1 teaspoon.

Salt

Pepper

Eggs, beaten - 2

Directions

Rinse the chicken tenders, pat dry.

In a medium bowl, pour in almond flour.

In a medium bowl, beat the eggs.

In a separate bowl, pour in almond meal. Season with rosemary, salt, pepper.

Take the chicken pieces and toast in flour, then egg, then almond meal. Set on a tray.

Place tray in freezer 5 minutes.

Preheat fryer to 350°F. Lightly spray cook basket with non-stick cooking spray.

Cook tenders 10 minutes. After the timer runs out, set temperature to 390°F, cook 5 more minutes until golden brown.

Serve on a platter. Side with preferred dipping sauce.

Nutritional info: Calories: 480, Fat: 36g, Carbs: 13g, Protein: 26g

Mahi-Mahi Tacos with Avocado and Fresh Cabbage

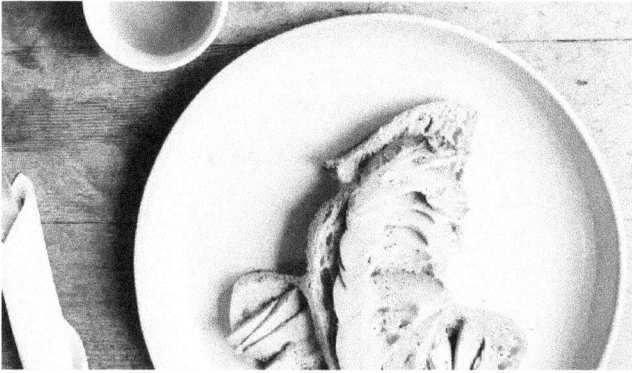

Preparation time: 5 minutes; Cook time: 15 minutes; Servings: 4

Ingredients:

Mahi-mahi - 1 pound.

Salt

Pepper

Olive oil - 1 teaspoon.

Avocado - 1

Corn tortillas - 4

Cabbage, shredded - 2 cups

Quartered limes – 2

Directions:

Season fish with salt and pepper.

Set a pan over medium-high heat. Add in oil and heat. Once the oil is hot, sauté fish for about 3–4 minutes on each side. Slice or flake fish into 1-ounce pieces.

Slice avocado in half. Remove seed and, using a spoon, remove the flesh from the skin. Slice the avocado halves into ½ thick slices.

In a small pan, warm corn tortillas; cook for about 1 minute on each side.

Place one-fourth of Mahi-mahi of each tortilla, top with avocado and cabbage. Serve with lime wedges.

Nutritional Info: Calories: 251, Fat: 9g, Protein: 25g, Carbs: 21g

Chapter 9:
Dinner

Pan-fried Jackfruit over Pasta with Lemon Coconut Cream Sauce

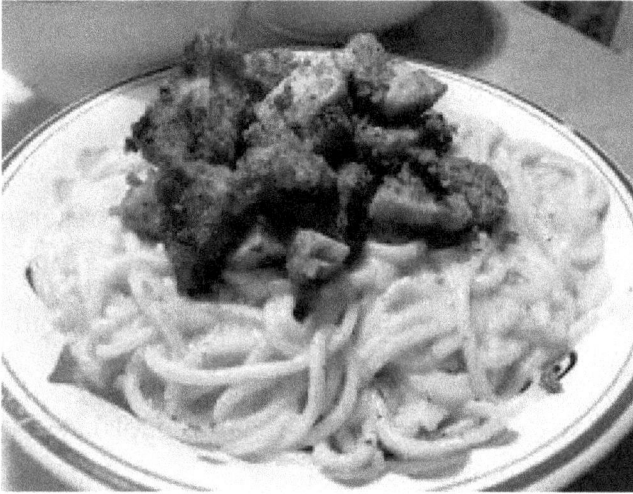

Preparation time: 5 minutes

Cooking time: 30 minutes

Servings: 6

Ingredients:

1 lb. pasta of choice

2 cans jackfruit in brine

2 tablespoons flour of choice

Garlic powder, dried oregano, paprika, black pepper, kosher salt to taste

2 tablespoons vegetable oil

4 tablespoons vegan butter

2 cups of coconut milk

Juice of 1 lemon

2 tablespoons grated vegan parmesan cheese

1 pinch ground nutmeg

1 teaspoon lemon zest (can use the same lemon from juice)

Fresh basil leaves, chopped for garnish

Directions

1. Cook pasta until al dente. Drain the pasta but reserve 1 cup of the pasta water. Set it aside for now.

2. While the pasta is cooking, drain the jackfruit and cut each piece in half. Pat jackfruit dry.

3. Mix flour with garlic powder, oregano, paprika, pepper, and salt in a separate bowl.

4. Toss flour mixture with jackfruit.

5. Heat vegetable oil in a skillet. Pan-fry the jackfruit until crisp on both sides. It takes around ten minutes in total.

6. Transfer the jackfruit to a plate lined with a paper towel and set aside.

7. In a large saucepan or skillet, melt vegan butter. Add coconut milk and lemon juice. Then add parmesan cheese and nutmeg. Cook until sauce is thick.

8. Add cooked pasta and half of the reserved pasta water to skillet. Toss to coat all pasta.

9. Cook until everything is hot and the sauce is to desired consistency and pasta is heated through. If the sauce is too thick, continue to use remaining pasta water.

10. Turn off heat. Add lemon zest and add pepper and salt to taste. Sprinkle parmesan and basil leaves. Add pan-fried jackfruit on top when serving.

Nutritional info: Calories: 480, Fat: 36g, Carbs: 13g, Protein: 26g

Butternut Squash Tacos with Tempeh Chorizo

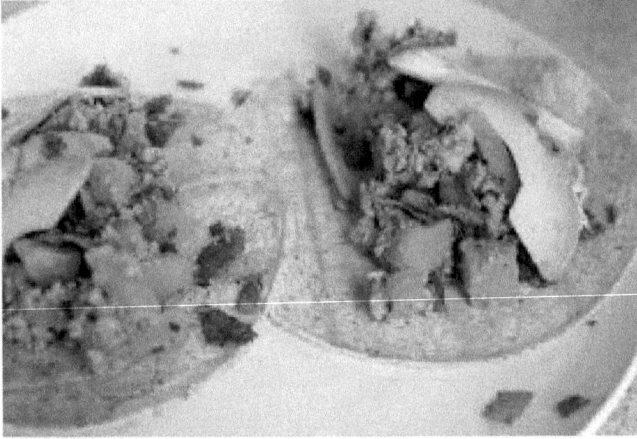

Preparation time: 5 minutes

Cooking time: 50 minutes

Servings: 5

Ingredients:

One 8-ounce package tempeh

½ cup of filtered water

¼ cup apple cider vinegar

2 cups butternut squash, peeled, cut into cubes

1 teaspoon chili powder

½ teaspoon smoked paprika

½ teaspoon cumin

½ teaspoon garlic powder

½ teaspoon oregano

A dash of cayenne

1 tablespoon nutritional yeast

A few dashes of liquid smoke

Black pepper and sea salt to taste

½ cup thinly julienned carrot (optional)

8 corn tortillas (or whatever you have on hand)

1 large avocado, pitted and sliced

Cilantro, chopped

Directions

1. Cut the tempeh into two parts. Steam for 10 min. Place in a large bowl and tear apart into small pieces either with your hands (after it's cooled) or with a pastry cutter.

2. While tempeh is steaming, bring water and vinegar to a boil in a small skillet.

3. Add spices, squash, liquid smoke, nutritional yeast, and a pinch of sea salt to skillet. Coat well and simmer covered, stirring occasionally. Add carrots and tempeh, covering again. Simmer a little while longer, stirring to prevent sticking. Uncover and season with pepper and salt.

4. Fill warmed tortillas with squash and tempeh mix and top with avocado and cilantro.

Nutritional info: Calories: 100, Fat: 36g, Carbs: 13g, Protein: 26g

Coated Cauliflower Head

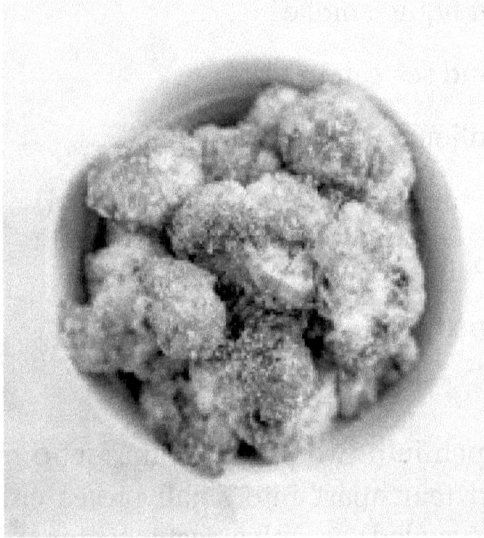

Preparation time: 10 minutes

Cooking time: 40 minutes

Servings:6

Ingredients:

2-pound cauliflower head

3 tablespoons olive oil

1 tablespoon butter, softened

1 teaspoon ground coriander

1 teaspoon salt

1 egg, whisked

1 teaspoon dried cilantro

1 teaspoon dried oregano

1 teaspoon tahini paste

Directions

Trim cauliflower head if needed.

Preheat oven to 350F.

In the mixing bowl, mix up together olive oil, softened butter, ground coriander, salt, whisked egg, dried cilantro, dried oregano, and tahini paste.

Then brush the cauliflower head with this mixture generously and transfer in the tray.

Bake the cauliflower head for 40 minutes.

Brush it with the remaining oil mixture every 10 minutes.

Nutritional info: Calories: 130, Fat: 10g, Carbs: 10g, Protein: 2g

Artichoke Petals Bites

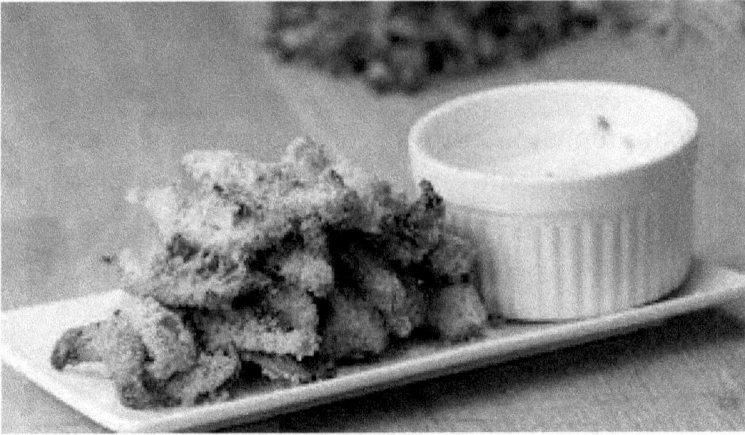

Preparation time: 10 minutes

Cooking time: 10 minutes

Servings:8

Ingredients:

8 oz artichoke petals, boiled, drained, without salt

½ cup almond flour

4 oz Parmesan, grated

2 tablespoons almond butter, melted

Directions

In the mixing bowl, mix up together almond flour and grated Parmesan.

Preheat the oven to 355F.

Dip the artichoke petals in the almond butter and then coat in the almond flour mixture.

Place them in the tray.

Transfer the tray in the preheated oven and cook the petals for 10 minutes.

Chill the cooked petal bites little before serving.

Nutritional info: Calories: 400, Fat: 36g, Carbs: 13g, Protein: 26g

Stuffed Beef Loin in Sticky Sauce

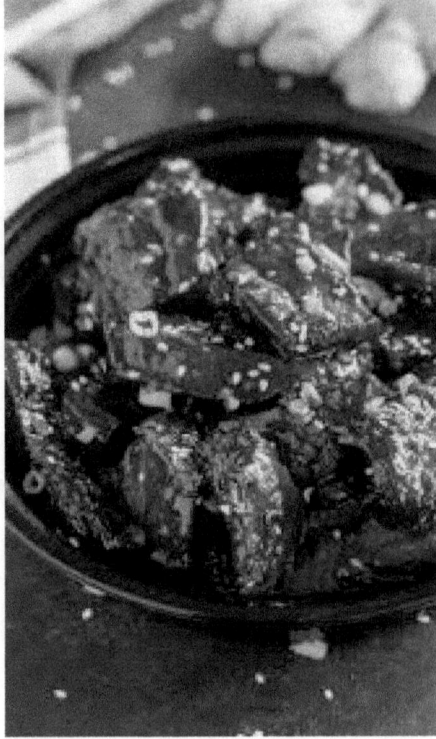

Preparation time: 15 minutes

Cooking time: 6 minutes

Servings:4

Ingredients:

1 tablespoon Erythritol

1 tablespoon lemon juice

4 tablespoons water

1 tablespoon butter

½ teaspoon tomato sauce

¼ teaspoon dried rosemary

9 oz beef loin

3 oz celery root, grated

3 oz bacon, sliced

1 tablespoon walnuts, chopped

¾ teaspoon garlic, diced

2 teaspoons butter

1 tablespoon olive oil

1 teaspoon salt

½ cup of water

Directions

Cut the beef loin into the layer and spread it with the dried rosemary, butter, and salt.

Then place over the beef loin: grated celery root, sliced bacon, walnuts, and diced garlic.

Roll the beef loin and brush it with olive oil.

Secure the meat with the help of the toothpicks.

Place it in the tray and add a ½ cup of water.

Cook the meat in the preheated to 365F oven for 40 minutes.

Meanwhile, make the sticky sauce: mix up together Erythritol, lemon juice, 4 tablespoons of water, and butter.

Preheat the mixture until it starts to boil.

Then add tomato sauce and whisk it well.

Bring the sauce to boil and remove from the heat.

When the beef loin is cooked, remove it from the oven and brush with the cooked sticky sauce very generously.

Slice the beef roll and sprinkle with the remaining sauce.

Nutritional info: Calories: 320, Fat: 26g, Carbs: 18g, Protein: 26g

Vegan Fish Sticks and Tartar Sauce

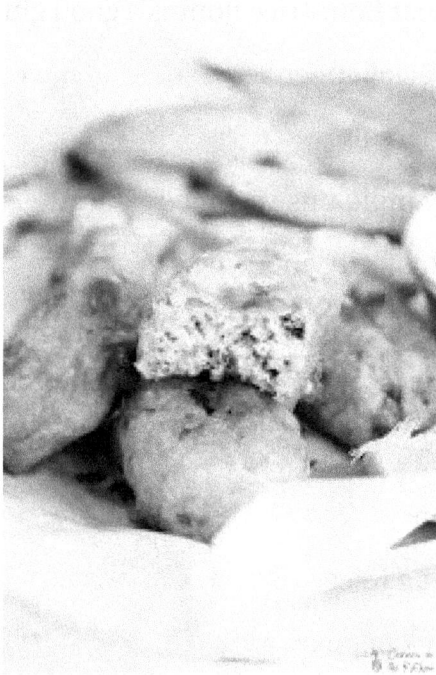

Preparation time: 5 minutes

Cooking time: 80 minutes

Servings: 6

Ingredients:

Fish Sticks:

12-ounce package extra-firm tofu

½ cup cornmeal

1 tablespoon garlic powder

1 tablespoon dried basil

2 tablespoons dulse flakes

1 tablespoon onion powder

½ cup whole wheat flour (rice flour is a good gluten-free option)

10 turns fresh black pepper

1 tablespoon of sea salt

¼ cup non-dairy milk, unsweetened

1 cup high-heat oil for frying

Vegan Tartar Sauce:

¼ cup sweet pickle relish

½ cup vegan mayo

½ teaspoon sugar

½ teaspoon lemon juice

5 turns fresh black pepper

Directions

1. Rinse tofu and drain in a colander. Placing a heavy plate on tofu with a heavy item on top will help drain better. Set it aside.

2. In a medium bowl, mix the flour, cornmeal, garlic powder, basil, onion powder, dulse flakes, pepper, and salt. Whisk together. Set the mix aside.

3. Set tofu on cutting board. Cut into quarters.

4. Slice tofu into thin pieces. You should have 28-32 pieces in total.

5. In a large cast-iron skillet, heat oil on medium/low heat.

6. In a small bowl, pour non-dairy milk.

7. Dip each piece of tofu in non-dairy milk. Immediately dip in breading, coating all sides evenly. Repeat until all pieces are coated.

8. The oil will start to splatter when hot enough. At that point, add tofu pieces to skillet. Repeat until all pieces are cooked.

9. Each side will cook for about 2-3 minutes. Watch for golden brown color. Place tofu pieces on a brown paper bag as you remove them from pan to soak up excess oil.

10. Repeat as necessary until all tofu is cooked. Cool before serving. Mix all tartar sauce ingredients until an even and creamy sauce is made. Enjoy!

Nutritional info: Calories: 480, Fat: 36g, Carbs: 13g, Protein: 26g

Vegan Philly Cheesesteak

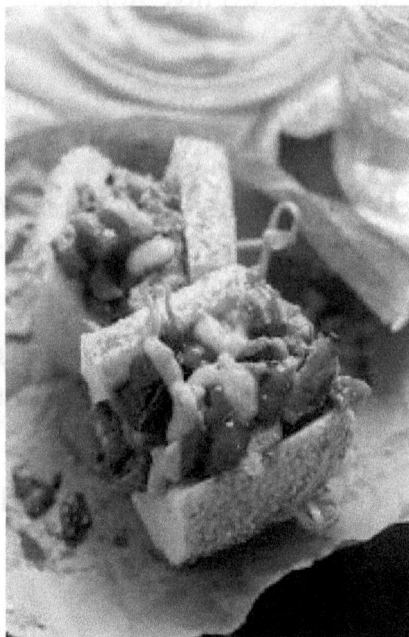

Preparation time: 5 minutes

Cooking time: 40 minutes

Servings: 4

Ingredients:

6-8 sliced Portobello mushrooms

4 cloves garlic, minced

1 tablespoon olive oil

1 whole clove garlic

½ teaspoon black pepper

1 teaspoon dried thyme

½ large diced onion

A dash of kosher salt

1 tablespoon vegan Worcestershire sauce

Hoagie rolls or another small loaf of bread of choice

1 cup shredded vegan cheddar cheese

Vegan mayo (optional)

Directions

1. Preheat the broiler.

2. In a deep skillet, heat olive oil. Brown mushrooms in oil, about 10 min.

3. Add thyme, garlic, and pepper until evenly coated.

4. Add onion and salt. Mushrooms must be well cooked before adding salt. Cook until onion is caramelized and softened, which should be for about 5 minutes. Add Worcestershire sauce and mix well.

5. Slice the bread lengthwise. Coat open sides of bread with olive oil or cooking spray. To add garlic flavor, cut the whole garlic clove, cut off the tip, and put on the oiled side of bread. Garlic powder is also a good substitute.

6. If desired, add optional vegan mayo. Place bread on cookie sheet. Fill loaves with mushrooms and top with shredded vegan cheddar cheese.

7. Place in broiler until cheese has melted, which should be 4-5 minutes.

Nutritional info: Calories: 123, Fat: 30g, Carbs: 10g, Protein: 20g

Pigs in a Blanket

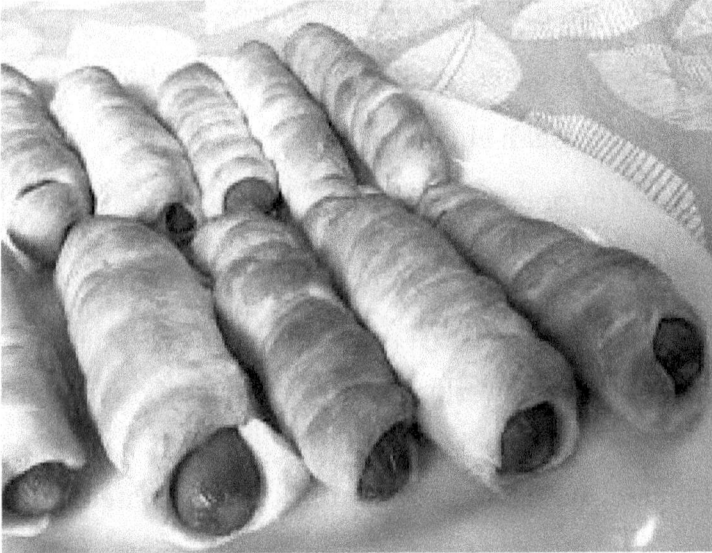

Preparation time: 5 minutes

Cooking time: 30 minutes

Servings: 6

Serves six

Ingredients:

Hot dogs, all-beef, twelve

Mozzarella cheese, shredded, two cups

Sesame seeds, one teaspoon

Eggs, two whisked

Coconut flour, one half cup

Cream cheese, two ounces at room temperature

Baking powder, one half teaspoon

Oregano, dried, one teaspoon

Garlic powder, one half teaspoon

Onion powder, one teaspoon

Directions

Heat oven to 400. Lay parchment paper on a cookie sheet. Put the cream cheese and mozzarella in a heatproof bowl and microwave for three minutes, then mix it together well until creamy. In another bowl mix together the eggs, baking powder, garlic powder, onion powder, oregano, and coconut flour until they are well mixed. Mix in the melted cheese. Wet your hands before sticking them in the dough because it will be sticky. Separate the dough into twelve equal-sized pieces and roll them into balls. Roll the balls of dough out into circles the same width as the hot dog is long. Roll up each hotdog with a circle of dough and lay them on the parchment paper on the cookie sheet. Sprinkle the sesame seeds on the dough and then bake for fifteen to twenty minutes until they are browned.

Nutrition per two hot dogs:

Calories 370, 7.5 grams net carbs, 23.5 grams fat, 24.5 grams protein

Baked Fish Sticks

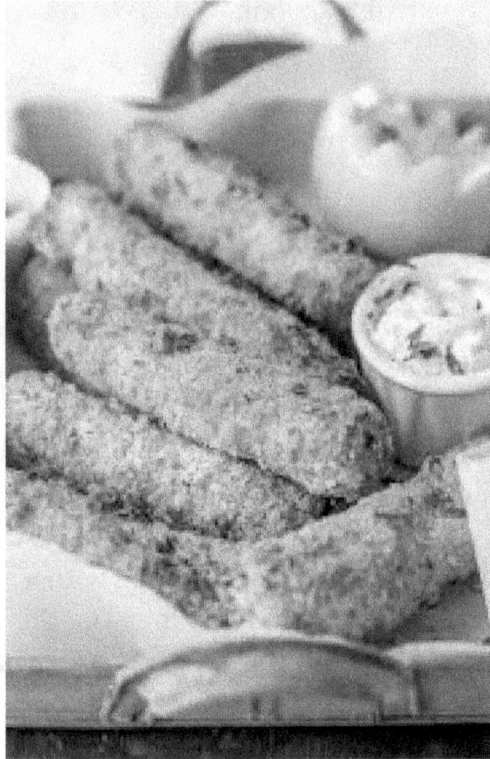

Preparation time: 5 minutes

Cooking time: 30 minutes

Servings: 6

Serves four

Ingredients:

Cod fillets, fresh, twelve ounces

Egg, one large

Pork rinds, one three and one half ounce bag

Coconut flour, one and one half tablespoons

Directions

Heat the oven to 400. Cut the codfish into strips and season them with the salt and pepper. Evenly coat the fish strips with the coconut flour. Smash the pork rinds into fine crumbs. Beat the water and egg white together well and use it to dip the fish strips into, and then into the pork rinds. Gently lay the fish sticks on a well-greased cookie sheet and bake them for fifteen minutes.

Nutrition per serving:

Calories 270, 1 gram net carbs, 11.5 grams fat, 38 grams protein

Lemon Parmesan Baked Cod

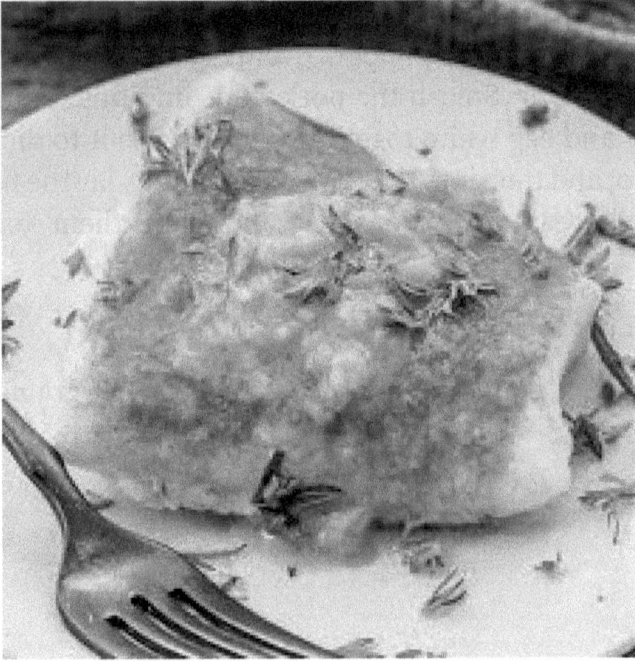

Serves four

Ingredients:

Cod fillets, boneless, two pounds

Lemon zest, one tablespoon

Parsley, chopped, one tablespoon

Paprika, one teaspoon

Parmesan cheese, grated, three-fourths cup

Garlic, minced, two tablespoons

Butter, melted, one quarter cup

Directions

Heat the oven to 400. Lay parchment paper over a cookie sheet. Cream together the garlic and butter in one bowl and mix the paprika with the parmesan in another bowl. Dip the fillets in the butter on both sides one by one and then roll them in the parmesan mixture. Lay the fillets on the cookie sheet. When all of the fillets are on the cookie sheet sprinkle them with the lemon zest and the parsley and bake for twenty minutes until the flesh of the fish separates easily with a fork.

Nutrition per serving:

Calories 320, 1 gram net carbs, 17.5 grams fat, 36.5 grams protein

Bacon-Wrapped Meatloaf

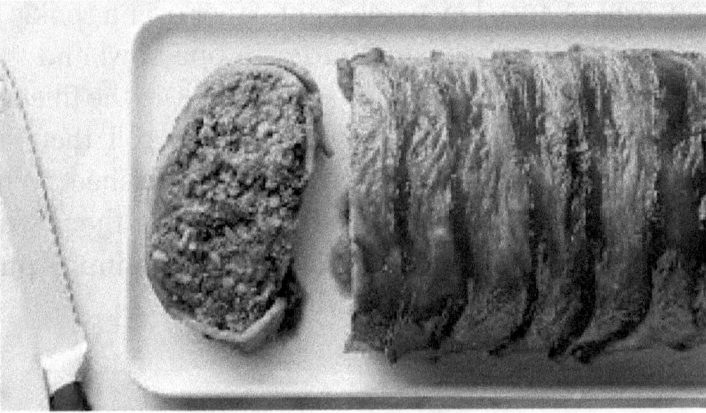

Preparation time: 5 minutes

Cooking time: 30 minutes

Servings: 6

Serves four

Ingredients:

Ground beef, two pounds

Egg, one

Cheddar cheese, shredded, one half cup

Heavy cream, for the gravy

Bacon, seven slices

Soy sauce, one tablespoon

Black pepper, one teaspoon

Salt, one teaspoon

Basil, dried one teaspoon

Oregano, dried, one teaspoon

Mayonnaise, one half cup

Yellow onion, one, chopped fine

Butter, two tablespoons

Directions

Heat the oven to 400. In the melted butter fry the onion for five minutes. Put the meat into a large bowl. Mix in the butter and onion mixture along with the remainder of the ingredients except for the bacon and the heavy cream. Use your hands to mix this together well, but do not overwork the mixture because this will make the meatloaf too dry. Use two tablespoons of lard to grease a nine-inch loaf dish. Make the meat mixture into a loaf shape and wrap the bacon around it. Bake for one hour. Remove the meat from the baking pan and pour the juices into a bowl with the whipping cream and mix well. Top the individual slices with the cream gravy mixture.

Nutrition per serving:

Calories 1038, 6 grams net carbs, 90 grams fat, 48 grams protein

Asian Meatballs with Basil Sauce

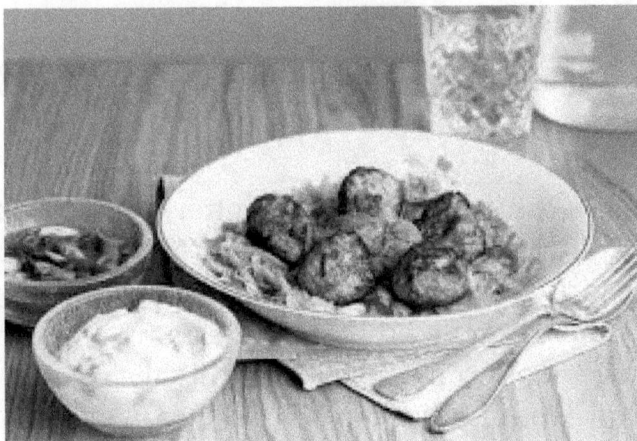

Preparation time: 5 minutes

Cooking time: 30 minutes

Servings: 6

Serves four

Ingredients:

ASIAN MEATBALLS

Ground pork, two pounds

Black pepper, one teaspoon

Ginger, ground, one tablespoon

Coconut oil, two tablespoons

Green cabbage, two cups shredded

Butter, two tablespoons

Yellow onion, minced, one half cup

BASIL SAUCE

Mayonnaise, three-fourths cup

Salt, one half teaspoon

Black pepper, one half teaspoon

Basil, fine chop, one tablespoon

Radishes, one half cup sliced paper-thin

PICKLED ONION SALAD

Rice vinegar, one tablespoon

Scallions, one ounce

Red chili pepper, one

Salt, one half teaspoon

Water, two tablespoons

Directions

MEATBALLS: Heat oven to 200. Mix well all of the ingredients for the meatballs using a large spoon or your hands. Shape this mix into twenty little meatballs. Fry the meatballs in hot coconut oil for ten minutes. Put the meatballs in the oven to keep them warm. Fry the green cabbage in the melted butter over medium heat in a large skillet for ten minutes, stirring it occasionally. Arrange the cabbage on a plate and lay the meatballs on top of the cabbage. Serve the onion salad and the basil sauce on the side.

PICKLED ONION SALAD: Slice the chili pepper and the scallions thinly and mix them with the rice vinegar, water, and salt and set this mix to the side.

BASIL SAUCE: Mix the sliced radishes with the basil and the mayonnaise. Add in the salt and the pepper, mix well and set this to the side.

Nutrition per serving:

Calories 860, 9 grams net carbs, 77 grams fat, 30 grams protein

Korma Curry

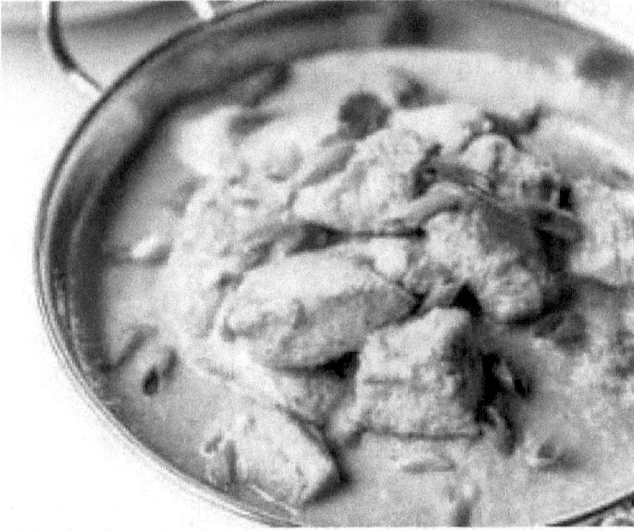

Preparation time: 10 minutes

Cooking time: 25 minutes

Servings: 6

Ingredients:

3-pound chicken breast, skinless, boneless

1 teaspoon garam masala

1 teaspoon curry powder

1 tablespoon apple cider vinegar

½ coconut cream

1 cup organic almond milk

1 teaspoon ground coriander

¾ teaspoon ground cardamom

½ teaspoon ginger powder

¼ teaspoon cayenne pepper

¾ teaspoon ground cinnamon

1 tomato, diced

1 teaspoon avocado oil

½ cup of water

Directions:

Chop the chicken breast and put it in the saucepan.

Add avocado oil and start to cook it over the medium heat.

Sprinkle the chicken with garam masala, curry powder, apple cider vinegar, ground coriander, cardamom, ginger powder, cayenne pepper, ground cinnamon, and diced tomato. Mix up the ingredients carefully. Cook them for 10 minutes.

Add water, coconut cream, and almond milk. Saute the meal for 10 minutes more.

Nutrition Values: calories 411, fat 19.3, fiber 0.9, carbs 6, protein 49.9

Zucchini Bars

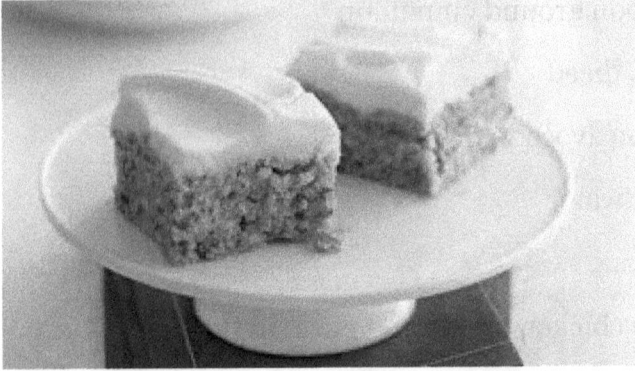

Preparation time: 10 minutes

Cooking time: 15 minutes

Servings: 8

Ingredients:

3 zucchini, grated

½ white onion, diced

2 teaspoons butter

3 eggs, whisked

4 tablespoons coconut flour

1 teaspoon salt

½ teaspoon ground black pepper

5 oz goat cheese, crumbled

4 oz Swiss cheese, shredded

½ cup spinach, chopped

1 teaspoon baking powder

½ teaspoon lemon juice

Directions:

In the mixing bowl, mix up together grated zucchini, diced onion, eggs, coconut flour, salt, ground black pepper, crumbled cheese, chopped spinach, baking powder, and lemon juice.

Add butter and churn the mixture until homogenous.

Line the baking dish with baking paper.

Transfer the zucchini mixture in the baking dish and flatten it.

Preheat the oven to 365F and put the dish inside.

Cook it for 15 minutes. Then chill the meal well.

Cut it into bars.

Nutrition Values: calories 199, fat 1316, fiber 215, carbs 7.1, protein 13.1

Mushroom Soup

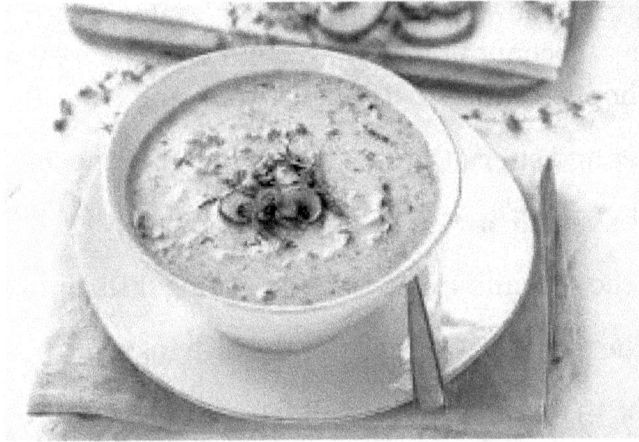

Preparation time: 10 minutes

Cooking time: 25 minutes

Servings: 4

Ingredients:

1 cup of water

1 cup of coconut milk

1 cup white mushrooms, chopped

½ carrot, chopped

¼ white onion, diced

1 tablespoon butter

2 oz turnip, chopped

1 teaspoon dried dill

½ teaspoon ground black pepper

¾ teaspoon smoked paprika

1 oz celery stalk, chopped

Directions:

Pour water and coconut milk in the saucepan. Bring the liquid to boil.

Add chopped mushrooms, carrot, and turnip. Close the lid and boil for 10 minutes.

Meanwhile, put butter in the skillet. Add diced onion. Sprinkle it with dill, ground black pepper, and smoked paprika. Roast the onion for 3 minutes.

Add the roasted onion in the soup mixture.

Then add chopped celery stalk. Close the lid.

Cook soup for 10 minutes.

Then ladle it into the serving bowls.

Nutrition Values: calories 181, fat 17.3, fiber 2.5, carbs 6.9, protein 2.4

Stuffed Portobello Mushrooms

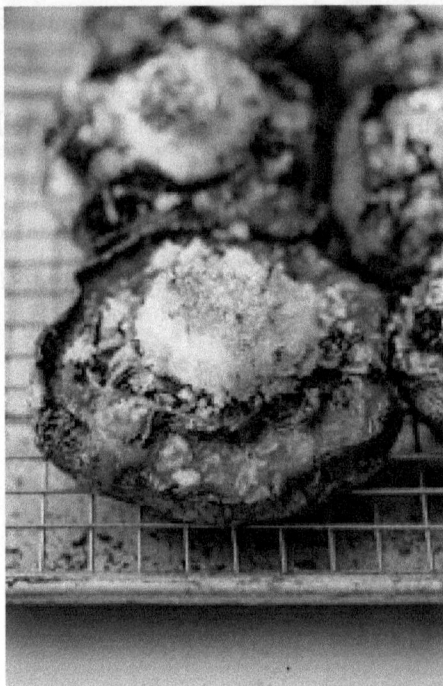

Preparation time: 10 minutes

Cooking time: 10 minutes

Servings: 4

Ingredients:

2 portobello mushrooms

1 cup spinach, chopped, steamed

2 oz artichoke hearts, drained, chopped

1 tablespoon coconut cream

1 tablespoon cream cheese

1 teaspoon minced garlic

1 tablespoon fresh cilantro, chopped

3 oz Cheddar cheese, grated

½ teaspoon ground black pepper

2 tablespoons olive oil

½ teaspoon salt

Directions:

Sprinkle mushrooms with olive oil and place in the tray.

Transfer the tray in the preheated to 360F oven and broil them for 5 minutes.

Meanwhile, blend together artichoke hearts, coconut cream, cream cheese, minced garlic, and chopped cilantro.

Add grated cheese in the mixture and sprinkle with ground black pepper and salt.

Fill the broiled mushrooms with the cheese mixture and cook them for 5 minutes more. Serve the mushrooms only hot.

Nutrition Values: calories 183, fat 16.3, fiber 1.9, carbs 3, protein 7.7

Lettuce Salad

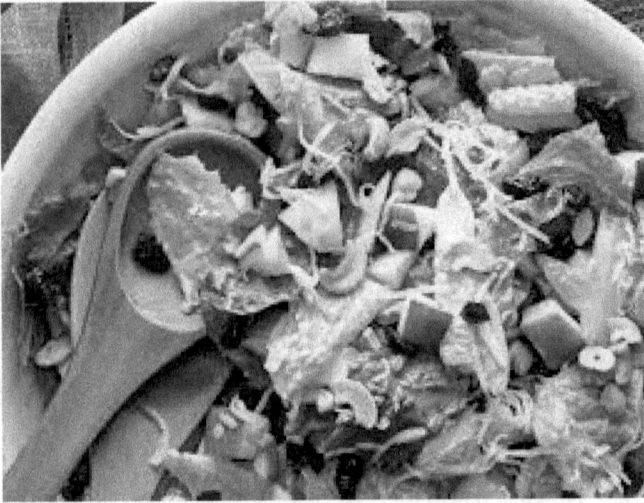

Preparation time: 10 minutes

Servings: 1

Ingredients:

1 cup Romaine lettuce, roughly chopped

3 oz seitan, chopped

1 tablespoon avocado oil

1 teaspoon sunflower seeds

1 teaspoon lemon juice

1 egg, boiled, peeled

2 oz Cheddar cheese, shredded

Directions:

Place lettuce in the salad bowl. Add chopped seitan and shredded cheese.

Then chop the egg roughly and add in the salad bowl too.

Mix up together lemon juice with the avocado oil.

Sprinkle the salad with the oil mixture and sunflower seeds. Don't stir the salad before serving.

Nutrition Values: calories 663, fat 29.5, fiber 4.7, carbs 3.8, protein 84.2

Onion Soup

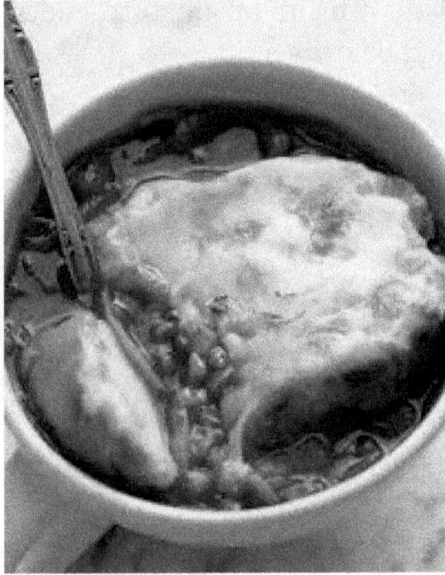

Preparation time: 10 minutes

Cooking time: 25 minutes

Servings: 6

Ingredients:

2 cups white onion, diced

4 tablespoon butter

½ cup white mushrooms, chopped

3 cups of water

1 cup heavy cream

1 teaspoon salt

1 teaspoon chili flakes

1 teaspoon garlic powder

Directions:

Put butter in the saucepan and melt it.

Add diced white onion, chili flakes, and garlic powder. Mix it up and saute for 10 minutes over the medium-low heat.

Then add water, heavy cream, and chopped mushrooms. Close the lid.

Cook the soup for 15 minutes more.

Then blend the soup until you get the creamy texture. Ladle it in the bowls.

Nutrition Values: calories 155, fat 15.1, fiber 0.9, carbs 4.7, protein 1.2

Asparagus Salad

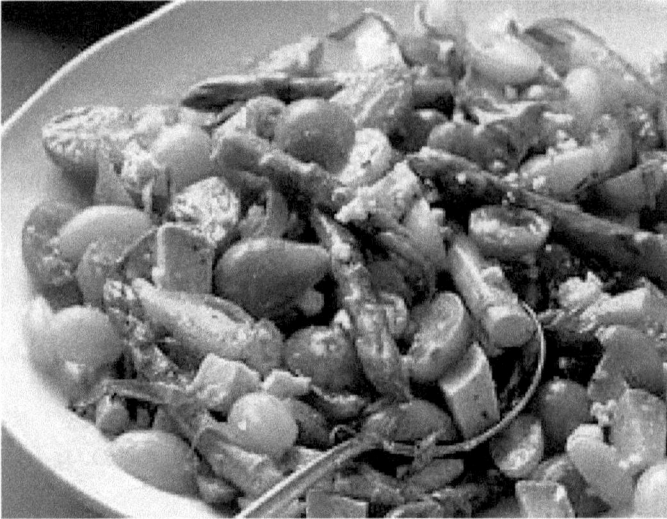

Preparation time: 10 minutes

Cooking time: 15 minutes

Servings: 3

Ingredients:

10 oz asparagus

1 tablespoon olive oil

½ teaspoon white pepper

4 oz Feta cheese, crumbled

1 cup lettuce, chopped

1 tablespoon canola oil

1 teaspoon apple cider vinegar

1 tomato, diced

Directions:

Preheat the oven to 365F.

Place asparagus in the tray, sprinkle with olive oil and white pepper and transfer in the preheated oven. Cook it for 15 minutes.

Meanwhile, put crumbled Feta in the salad bowl.

Add chopped lettuce and diced tomato.

Sprinkle the ingredients with apple cider vinegar.

Chill the cooked asparagus to the room temperature and add in the salad.

Shake the salad gently before serving.

Nutrition Values: calories 207, fat 17.6, fiber 2.4, carbs 6.8, protein 7.8

Chapter 10:
4 Weeks Meal plan

DAYS	BREAKFAST	LUNCH	DINNER
1	Zucchini Omelet	Vegan Tuna Salad	Pan-fried Jackfruit over Pasta with Lemon Coconut Cream Sauce
2	Chili Omelet	Veggie Wrap with Apples and Spicy Hummus	Butternut Squash Tacos with Tempeh Chorizo
3	Basil and Cherry Tomato Breakfast	Turmeric Rack of Lamb	Coated Cauliflower Head
4	Carrot Breakfast Salad	Sausage Casserole	Artichoke Petals Bites
5	Garlic Zucchini Mix	Cajun Pork Sliders	Stuffed Beef Loin in Sticky Sauce
6	Crustless Broccoli Sun-dried Tomato Quiche	Mac and Cheese Bites	Vegan Fish Sticks and Tartar Sauce
7	Chocolate Pancakes	Chick'n Salad with Cranberries and Pistachios	Vegan Philly Cheesesteak
8	Breakfast Scramble	Tuna Casserole	Pigs in a Blanket
9	Oatmeal	White Fish with Curry and Coconut	Baked Fish Sticks

10	Coconut Cream with Berries	Creamy Fish Casserole	Lemon Parmesan Baked Cod
11	Seafood Omelet	Spinach and Goat Cheese Pie	Bacon-Wrapped Meatloaf
12	Spinach and Pork with Fried Eggs	Avocado Pie	Asian Meatballs with Basil Sauce
13	Smoked Salmon Sandwich	Tex Mex Stuffed Zucchini Boats	Korma Curry
14	Shrimp Deviled Eggs	Brussel Sprouts and Hamburger Gratin	Zucchini Bars
15	Scrambled Eggs with Halloumi Cheese	SoyLime Roasted Tofu	Mushroom Soup
16	Coconut Porridge	Chicken Nuggets	Stuffed Portobello Mushrooms
17	Western Omelet	Crab-Stuffed Avocado	Lettuce Salad
18	Mushroom Omelet	Thai Fish Curry	Onion Soup
19	Frittata with Fresh Spinach	Avocado Grapefruit Salad	Asparagus Salad
20	Cauliflower Hash Browns	Garlic Herb Grilled Chicken Breast	Coated Cauliflower Head
21	Salmon Filled Avocado	Cajun Shrimp	Artichoke Petals Bites
22	Rutabaga Fritters with Avocado	Sesame-Crusted Mahi-Mahi	Stuffed Beef Loin in Sticky Sauce

23	Bacon Mushroom Breakfast Casserole	Country Chicken	Vegan Fish Sticks and Tartar Sauce
24	Baked Eggs	Mahi-Mahi Tacos with Avocado and Fresh Cabbage	Vegan Philly Cheesesteak
25	Keto Blueberry Muffins	Tuna Casserole	Pigs in a Blanket
26	Taco Breakfast Skillet	Turmeric Rack of Lamb	Baked Fish Sticks
27	Cream Cheese Pancakes	Mac and Cheese Bites	Lemon Parmesan Baked Cod
28	Keto Cloud Bread	White Fish with Curry and Coconut	Bacon-Wrapped Meatloaf

Conclusion

Thank you for making it through to the end of this book. After being exposed to so much knowledge about intermittent fasting, you aren't likely to be surprised by the fact that the American Heart Association recommends intermittent fasting for losing weight. Its effectiveness in helping women lose weight is backed by science as well as by the personal experiences of thousands of women.

Fasting has existed in religious traditions for millennia, and now anyone can harness its health benefits with intermittent fasting. You don't have to undergo nearly the level of physical and mental fatigue of traditional water fasts, but you still see the difference in your waistline and in how you feel.

The scientific credibility that intermittent fasting has is all thanks to the biological process of autophagy. Autophagy is your body's natural means of getting rid of toxins that pollute your system. Intermittent fasting is your means of triggering this vital process.

Intermittent fasting is your ticket into triggering autophagy because it is easy to sustain. Unlike other means of achieving autophagy, intermittent fasting doesn't ask that you go to the gym or change what you eat (although you should still these things to get the most out of the biological process). Start your intermittent fast today and you will see all the health benefits uncovered in this book for yourself.

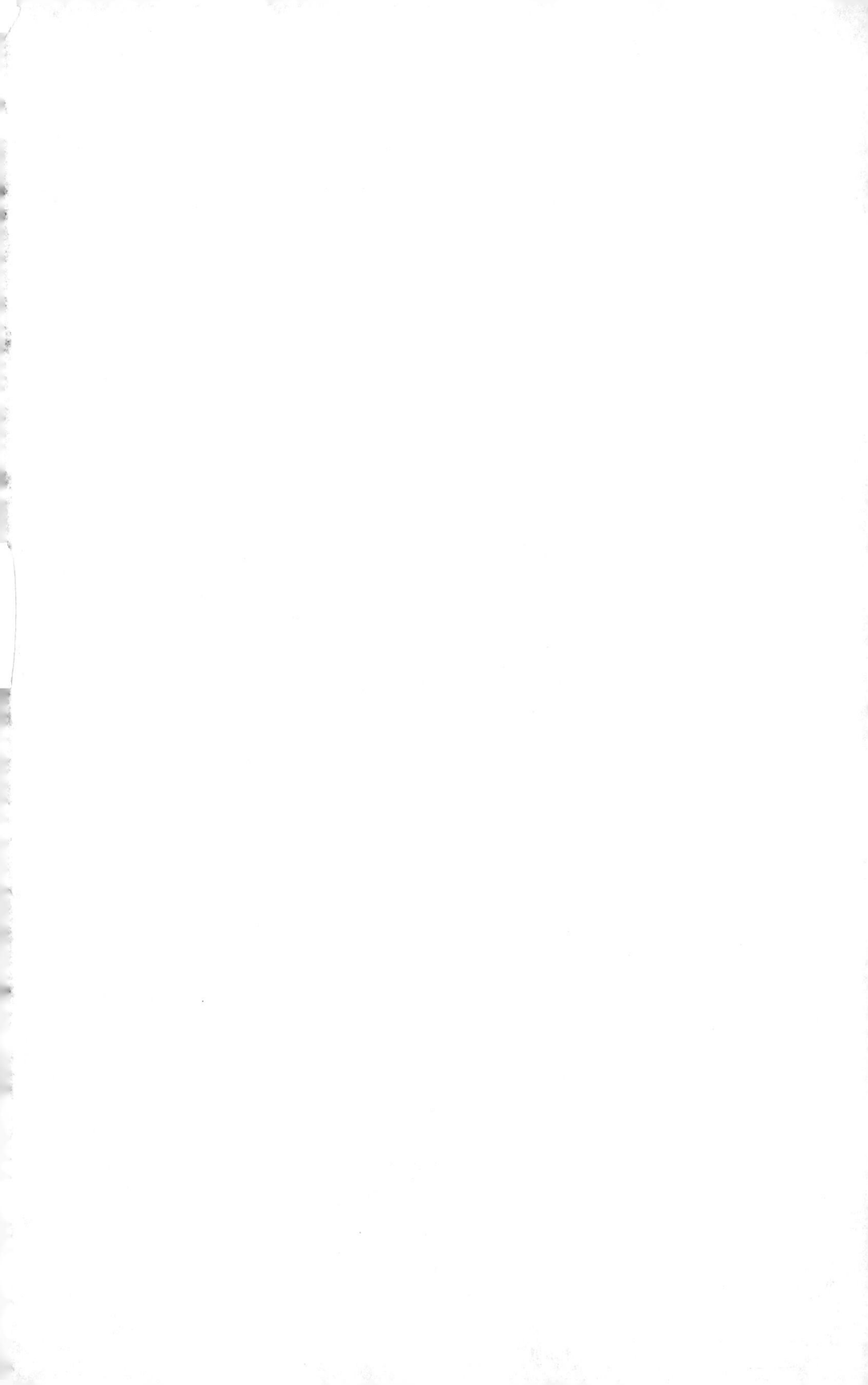